A Brief Guide to the

NEURORADIOLOGY FELLOWSHIP

Online Resources

High-Yield Learning Resources with Links:

https://tinyurl.com/neurorad-resources

Efficiency-Oriented Macro Library:

https://tinyurl.com/neurorad-macros

A Brief Guide to the

NEURORADIOLOGY

FELLOWSHIP

LONG H. TU MD

Neuroradiology Fellow 2020-2021
Yale New Haven Hospital,
New Haven, CT, USA

ISBN: 9798524122469

Disclaimer

Every effort has been made in preparing this book to provide accurate information in accordance to policies and practice at the time of publication. Nevertheless, the authors, editors and publishers can make no warranties that the information contained herein is totally free from error, not least because clinical standards are constantly changing through research and regulation.

The authors, editors, and publishers therefore disclaim all liability for direct or consequential damages resulting from the use of material contained in this book.

For my family.

Preface & Guidelines for Use

Neuroradiology has historically been the most popular subspecialty in radiology, accounting for 15-20% of all graduates from US residency programs. Like the broader radiology training pool, fellows have a diverse set of career goals, spanning private, mixed, and traditionally academic practice. The preparation for subspecialty training is variable across residencies, and the depth and complexity of neuroradiology can be overwhelming for even the most confident trainees. Using all of the recommended textbooks, questions banks, and other resources available to residents still cannot prepare a trainee fully for what is to come. This is because there are gaps in what is identified as essential understanding prior to the beginning of fellowship.

Subspecialty neuroradiology requires familiarity with exams and procedures that residents may not have not seen with significant frequency (e.g., MRI brachial/lumbar plexus, MRI of the fetus, MR spectroscopy, and fMRI). For programs that require fellows take acute "neuro call" shortly after starting, the beginning of fellowship can unexpectedly present the steepest and highest stakes learning curve encountered during the whole of radiology training.

The goal of this manual is not to recapitulate what is well-written elsewhere on the neuroradiology knowledge base. Instead, the aims are to 1) organize underappreciated resources into a *strategy guide* for learning – with an emphasis on preparation for call 2) provide high-yield, yet-unwritten notes on workflow, blind spots, and search patterns for uncommon exams, and 3) accomplish the aforementioned using as few words as possible.

In the interest of brevity, I will assume a familiarity with all common radiologic terms, anatomy, pathology, and physics up to the level of a senior resident. I'll presume an ability to look up images, review articles, and other resources as needed. In the interest of making the text as broadly applicable as possible, I've focused the topics on issues and radiologic studies that may not be seen by residents commonly, but will apply to *most* fellowship programs. Extremely uncommon and rare exam types are not discussed. Even some of the studies discussed in the sections on search patterns may not apply to all practice settings. Please feel free to skip topics as convenient.

This book is not meant to be read cover to cover. The sections on learning strategy and resources might best be approached either prior to fellowship or immediately after starting. Tips on workflow and efficiency, common errors, and acute/vascular exams would also likely pay greatest dividends in the early months. Specific search patterns and checklists for procedures or advanced exams could be referenced as needed. These sections might best be reviewed real time, at the workstation.

This book is written in an informal style and published independently to maximize the speed and accessibility of communication. Please excuse any undetected typos and other (hopefully small!) flaws. I encourage you to check any unclear information with trusted resources. I should also mention that while I recruited numerous collaborators, every expressed opinion is my own, as I had complete creative control over this work. The thoughts contained herein do not necessarily reflect the views of my co-authors, institution, or other affiliates.

In summary, this is a collection of practical wisdom that I couldn't find written down anywhere else. It is what I would pass on to every new fellow, if only I had the time to sit down to do it for each person. I hope you'll find the resulting book to be a useful tool in your journey in becoming a great neuroradiologist and physician.

Long H. Tu
6/30/2021

"I am a brain, Watson.

The rest of me is a mere appendix."

- Arthur Conan Doyle

Table of Contents

Introduction **v**
Preface & Guidelines for Use vi
Acknowledgements xi
Contributors xiii

High-Yield Learning Resources **1**
Assumed Knowledge Base Prior to Fellowship 2
Late Residency & Early Fellowship 3
Middle to Late Fellowship 4
Video Resources 4
Book Recommendations 5
Highest Yield Review Articles 7
Additional Curated Review Articles 11

Dictation Efficiency and Macros **14**
Dictate to Guide Management, Not to Enumerate Abnormality 15
Maximize Macro-Based Efficiency 17
Prioritize Safety and Continuous Improvement Over Perfection 20
Shared Macro Library Link 21

Common Errors on Neuroimaging Studies **22**
General Workflow and Habits 24
Non-Contrast CT Head 30
CT Neck Notes 32
CTA Head and Neck 34
MRI Brain 40
CT/MRI Orbits Notes 44
MRI Spine Studies 45

Search Patterns for Acute/Vascular Exams **48**
MRA Brain 49
Vessel Wall Imaging 52
MRA Neck 55
MRV Brain 58
CT Perfusion for Stroke 62
MR Perfusion for Stroke 65

Search Patterns for Uncommon MRI Exams **68**
MRI Brachial Plexus 69
MRI Thoracic Outlet Syndrome 74
MRI Lumbosacral Plexus 77
MRI Temporomandibular Joints 82
MRI Fetus for CNS Abnormalities 86

Search Patterns for Uncommon CT Studies **92**
4D CT for Parathyroid Adenomas 93
CT Conebeam Maxillofacial Notes 98
Dual Energy CT Head 104

Checklists for Advanced MRI **107**
Functional MRI (fMRI) 108
MR Spectroscopy (MRS) 116
MR Perfusion for Tumor 121

Checklists and Tips for Common Procedures **127**
Fluoroscopy Guided Lumbar Puncture 129
Lumbar Epidural Injection 136
Epidural Blood Patch 139
CT Myelogram 143
CT Guided Spine/Soft Tissue Biopsy 146

Workflow and Team Efficiency Tips **152**
Communication Triage and Automation 153
Protocoling Automation and Efficiency 155
Differentiation of Administrative Roles 156
Teaching and Academics 157

Conclusion **xiv**
Last Comments & Contact xv

Acknowledgements

It has been a challenging though satisfying year. This book and my wellbeing during the time of its writing I credit to my closest friends and family. Thank you especially to Vince, Tom, Alice, Yari, and Rebecca for always being there for me.

Fellowship has been an intensely engaging and humbling time. That it's also been a good experience, I owe to the dedication of our program director Bill Zucconi and associate program director Anthony Abou Karam. What a challenge to have started in the midst of a pandemic. You were both unbelievably supportive and flexible as we figured out how to be fellows in unprecedented circumstances.

I am perhaps most lucky to work closely with my once again co-chief, Reid Kraniski, who is the most amazing teammate I could have asked for. I hope any positive impact we had will propagate forward in the years to come. It has been a special privilege to work closely with you these past years.

A great thanks to David Homa and Betty Mathew, who helped smooth our start at the end of their off-cycle year.

And then to the people (co-fellows and friends) who made year not just doable but also fun... Thanks to Mehmet and Brooke for a great year. I am so happy you're sticking around! Thank you, Jerry and Lenny, for being especially kind and always great team players. Junaid, thank you for passing on life lessons and being so flexible. Sarvenaz and Jesus, I can't we made it this far since that first meeting in Hewitt. I will see you again soon! Nakul, I'm so happy you were a part of our team. Neuro was always the right choice! Allen – it was a privilege to share so many early shifts with you. You taught me a lot about life and radiology. Andrea, our next class could not be luckier in having your early guidance.

Bilal (and Andrea), thank you so much to taking lead on organizational needs at the end of the year. This book would not be released on time without your help on that front!

And thank you Emily. The procedure service feels like a disaster without you and the best run rotation when you're there.

I must again credit the infamous and unparalleled Prometheus Lionhart, who set the precedent for independent writing and publishing in our field. Your shepherding of the first of my books laid the groundwork for this next, more focused volume. Our specialty, and medical practice by extension, is much better off because your efforts.

I owe a great debt to my mentor Howard ("Howie") Forman for being a guiding light for the past few years. You have been incredibly kind, patient, and thoughtful in helping me grapple with all manner of both career and personal challenges.

I would also not be here without the numerous engaged and amazing teachers I had in both residency and fellowship. I must mention at least my former program director, S. A. Jamal Bokhari, whose vision and support convinced me that maybe more is possible than we can begin to imagine – I have tried to live up to that hope and am here in large part because of it.

This book was made much better through the time, effort, and vision of my co-authors. They are listed at beginning of each relevant chapter and also together on the following page. Among these, I have to give particular gratitude to Sandra Abi Fadel, who rushed to help on sections where I didn't know how to go forward. And lastly, Ichiro Ikuta, whose feedback and encouragement planted the seed of this book. This would not have been possible without you.

Thank you all!

Contributors

Sandra Abi Fadel, MD
Assistant Professor of Radiology
Section of Neuroradiology
Yale School of Medicine
Yale-New Haven Hospital

Mariam Aboian, MD PhD
Assistant Professor of Radiology
Section of Neuroradiology
Yale School of Medicine
Yale-New Haven Hospital

Anthony Abou Karam, MD
Assistant Professor of Radiology
Section of Neuroradiology
Yale School of Medicine
Yale-New Haven Hospital

Mehmet Emin Adin, MD
Clinical Fellow
Section of Neuroradiology
Yale School of Medicine
Yale-New Haven Hospital

Ichiro Ikuta, MD MMSc
Assistant Professor of Radiology
Section of Neuroradiology
Yale School of Medicine
Yale-New Haven Hospital

Michele Johnson, MD
Professor of Radiology
Section of Neuroradiology
Yale School of Medicine
Yale-New Haven Hospital

Amit Mahajan, MD
Assistant Professor of Radiology
Section of Neuroradiology
Yale School of Medicine
Yale-New Haven Hospital

Sam Payabvash, MD
Assistant Professor of Radiology
Section of Neuroradiology
Yale School of Medicine
Yale-New Haven Hospital

Balaji Rao, MBBCh
Assistant Professor of Radiology
Section of Neuroradiology
Yale School of Medicine
Yale-New Haven Hospital

Kimberly Seifert, MD
Clinical Fellow
Diagnostic Neuroradiology
Stanford School of Medicine
Stanford Medicine

Elizabeth Schrickel, MD
Clinical Fellow
Section of Neuroradiology
Yale School of Medicine
Yale-New Haven Hospital

William Zucconi, DO
Associate Professor of Radiology
Section of Neuroradiology
Yale School of Medicine
Yale-New Haven Hospital

High-Yield Learning Resources

Long H. Tu

Elizabeth Brooke Schrickel

William Zucconi

Introduction

It is hard to find guidance on how best to approach independent learning during the fellowship year. The ASNR publishes a curriculum, which encompasses a list of relevant topics, rather than a set of resources or a roadmap. There is not a set of consensus core texts as there may be for residency. For those who prefer a global/top-down view of the field, this can lead to some disorientation as to where to start and what to prioritize.

What follows is a best effort at consolidating available resources, insight from recent trainees, fellowship directors, and personal experience into a learning strategy. I'm discussing resources specifically with regard to the more common one-year fellowship structure, though the approach could be modified for other tracks. The usual caveats apply that this mostly consists of collected opinions and experience.

Please note that this chapter is available as a web-based document with embedded links here: https://tinyurl.com/neurorad-resources.

Assumed Knowledge Base Prior to Fellowship

To make fellowship level recommendations, I have to assume a certain knowledge base. The following are the "consensus" resources used by trainees across the nation to build a knowledge base in neuroradiology *prior* to fellowship. I'm going to assume coverage of most/all of these (consider filling in any gaps at the end of residency if needed):

- *Core Radiology* by Jacob Mandel (neuroradiology chapter)
- *Crack the Core* by Prometheus Leonhart (neuroradiology sections)
- *Neuroradiology: A Core Review* by Dubey et al
- RADPrimer Question Bank (neuroradiology questions)
- *Neuroradiology Companion* by Mauricio Castillo
- *Duke Review of MRI Physics: Case Review Series* by Mangrum et al
- https://radiologyassistant.nl/neuroradiology

The following texts are also sometimes used by residents, but I can tell you that they are somewhat redundant with the above. These could be skipped if you've done most of the preceding:

- *Neuroradiology: The Requisites* by Nadgir and Yousem
- *Brant and Helms' Fundamentals of Diagnostic Radiology* by Klein et al
- *Textbook of Radiology and Imaging* by Sutton

Late Residency & Early Fellowship

At the beginning of fellowship, it is essential to get a refresher on topics in acute/emergency neuroimaging, and if possible, cover a broad set of topics that can get you oriented to routine studies.

For the first of these tasks, two resources stand out, the publicly available *2019 RadioGraphics Monograph Issue: Emergency Neuroradiology* and the beginning chapters of *Osborn's Brain* (the book), which are focused on emergency neuroimaging. These overlap to some degree, and some material will be familiar from residency. If I had to pick one, I'd go with the former; though if you end up using both, you can just skim areas of overlap. For those with deeper interest, there is *Emergency Neuroradiology: A Case-Based Approach* by Tang et al. It's very easy to flip through quickly.

For an introduction to neuroradiology at the fellow level, I highly recommend the publicly available *ASNR Neurocurriculum Live video series.* It is useful to focus on emergent or unfamiliar topics first. The series is approximately 80 videos, most <15mins. In the Chrome web browser however, you can get a plug-in (Video Speed Controller) that speeds up embedded videos. This can reduce the total watch time to <10 hours. The topics I'd do in early fellowship account for probably less than 2 hours total.

Other curated articles and videos are listed below, focused on topics that will help you with exam types and topics not commonly seen on at the resident level. Consider reading these (or others on the same topic) early in the year.

Summary of Resources for Early Fellowship

- Recommend at least ONE of the following, not necessarily all:
    - "2019 RadioGraphics Monograph Issue: Emergency Neuroradiology"
    - Osborn's Brain by Osborn et al (the ~1300 page of the two versions, first chapters on emergency topics).
    - *Emergency Neuroradiology: A Case-Based Approach* by Tang
    - "ASNR Fellow Education: Neurocurriculum Live video series" - can be watched sped up for efficiency with plugin. Focus on emergency/unfamiliar topics first.

- High yield review articles for early fellowship on acute and possibly unfamiliar topics.
    - CT/MR perfusion for stroke:
        - Wing, Stevan Christopher, and Hugh S. Markus. **"Interpreting CT perfusion in stroke."** Practical neurology 19.2 (2019): 136-142.
        - Demeestere, Jelle, et al. **"Review of perfusion imaging in acute ischemic stroke: from time to tissue."** Stroke 51.3 (2020): 1017-1024.
    - Teeth/Dental Emergencies:
        - Loureiro, Rafael M., et al. **"Dental emergencies: a practical guide."** Radiographics 39.6 (2019): 1782-1795. (in the 2019 RadioGraphics Monograph Issue)
        - Scheinfeld, Meir H., et al. **"Teeth: what radiologists should know."** Radiographics 32.7 (2012): 1927-1944.

Middle to Late Fellowship

The problem with neuroradiology is how vast the knowledge base is required to practice at a high level across all subdomains. Brain, spine, head and neck, pediatric neuroradiology, and interventional neuroradiology could each stand on their own as separate fields given the size of the knowledge base. When I started fellowship, it was not clear from the advice I got whether you *had* to read anything comprehensive at all. Depending on whether you like reading books or not, there are a few approaches to getting an overview, which I'll detail below.

Video Resources

I would recommend completing *all* of the ASNR Neurocurriculum Live video series for basically all fellows. There are also video lecture series produced in review courses by some major academic centers (Mass Gen, Penn, Duke). These could be use as supplements, though are not publicly available. YouTube also has great teaching videos. Many academic departments provide free teaching videos. A curated list of high-yield videos is provided below.

- "ASNR Fellow Education: Neurocurriculum Live video series" - can be watched sped up for efficiency with plugin.
- Review Courses (Mass Gen, Penn, Duke), which may be purchased/available through your program.
- Curated YouTube lecture series:
  - Yale Neuroradiology Videos by Dr. Leon Kier: https://youtube.com/playlist?list=PLMoHC7ioYlMYqJDVNuoIDFIksoTFJwU6b
  - ASHNR webinar series on Youtube. Specifically, this lecture by Drs Pat Rhyner and Ashley Aiken on Cancer staging of the Head and Neck. https://youtu.be/U90aSKUIAX8
  - Learn Neuroradiology Youtube Channel by Dr. Brent Weinberg: https://learnneuroradiology.com/tag/videos/
  - Michigan State University Department of radiology Head and Neck Lectures: https://youtube.com/playlist?list=PLovbk6NLAFAtJWzYUhnnp6kdRRYct7gOr

Book Recommendations

If there is only one conventional book that I would recommend fellows read, it is the most recent edition of *Osborne's Brain*. It can be a little intimidating at ~1300 pages, but is extremely readable. There's a lot of pictures and some clinical/genetic/other information you can just gloss over, while focusing on the imaging. If you aim for 30-50 "pages" per day, five days a week, you can be done with Osborne's Brain in 1-2 months. Very doable for the first part of fellowship.

Reading books beyond Osborn's Brain is not as high yield, though still worthwhile for those who like physical texts. For head and neck, the most approachable/readable is *Head and Neck Imaging: Case Series* by Yousem. There are a few reference texts by Som and Mancuso and others, which are a bit expensive and >2000-3000 pages. These might best used as reference (or sub-subspecialty training) for when a deep dive is necessary.

There are a few book options for spine. *Spine Imaging: Case Review Series* by Saraf-Lavi and *Spine Imaging: A Case-Based Guide to Imaging and Management* by Gupta et al and are the most approachable. The first of these may require some real-time look up and fact checking, though is on balance a more interesting and advanced read. It is worth your time if you like books and are willing to put in the time.

You probably do not need to read a specific book for pediatric neuroradiology. *Pediatric Neuroradiology* by Choudhri is probably the most approachable standalone text, but is very introductory, and does not add much if you've already done the other resources. The famous *Pediatric Neuroimaging* by Barkovich is very detailed and not as amenable to a straight readthrough; it is best used as a reference in deeper sub-subspecialty training. *Osborn's Brain* covers pediatric neuroradiology to a practical degree, and may suffice for almost all needs outside very specialized centers. You could also read nothing beyond focused review articles in this area as needed.

For angiography, an outstanding reference is the *Neuroangio.org* website by Maksim Shapiro. This is probably too extensive to read entirely as part of a single year curriculum, though could be perused for reference as needed. High-yield review articles for other neuroradiology procedures are listed at the end of this chapter as well as associated with corresponding checklists in later chapters.

Summary of Recommended Books (for the reading-oriented):

- **Brain:** *Osborn's Brain* by Osborn et al – A highly recommend read if you had to choose one.
- **Head and neck:** *Head and Neck Imaging: Case Series* by Yousem (optional).
- **Spine:** *Spine Imaging: Case Review Series* by Saraf-Lavi OR *Spine Imaging: A Case-Based Guide to Imaging and Management* by Gupta et al (both optional).
- **Pediatric:** Relevant chapters in *Osborn's Brain* OR *Pediatric Neuroradiology* by Choudhri (both optional).

- Texts that are great references, though not as amenable to a cover-to-cover read:
    - *Problem Solving in Neuroradiology* by Law et al – Some sections are very good (especially those on MR perfusion and MR spectroscopy), though the Neurocurriculum live lectures and later referenced articles cover this well also.
    - The *Diagnostic Imaging* Series – A reproduction of StatDx onto physical paper. The books are beautiful, but are very

expensive, and less approachable from a reading cover-to-cover perspective. I would recommend just using StatDx if you have it.

- *Magnetic Resonance Imaging of the Brain and Spine* by Atlas – A nice reference outside of brain sections (for which Osborn's Brain is more accessible).
- *Head and Neck Imaging* by Som and Curtin – Very detailed. Best as a reference.
- *Head and Neck Radiology* by Mancuso – Very detailed. Best as a reference.
- *Pediatric Neuroimaging* by Barkovich – The chapters on brain and spine injury, which cover ischemia and infarcts are excellent for the interested.

Highest Yield Review Articles

There are a few articles that cover topics highly relevant to all neuroradiologists that are not covered in depth by many texts. Many of these (especially those associated with an uncommon exam types) are also referenced in associated chapters later on in this book. Below is a curated short list by topic. They are ordered roughly in suggested order of priority.

- Efficient Reporting:
  - Hartung MP, Bickle IC, Gaillard F, Kanne JP. **How to Create a Great Radiology Report**. RadioGraphics. 2020 Oct;40(6):1658-70.

- Perfusion Imaging for Stroke:
  - Heit JJ, Wintermark M. **Perfusion computed tomography for the evaluation of acute ischemic stroke: strengths and pitfalls.** Stroke. 2016 Apr;47(4):1153-8.

- Essential White Papers on Incidental Findings:
  - Hoang, J.K., Hoffman, A.R., González, R.G., Wintermark, M., Glenn, B.J., Pandharipande, P.V., Berland, L.L. and Seidenwurm, D.J., 2018. **Management of incidental pituitary findings on CT, MRI, and 18F-**

fluorodeoxyglucose PET: A white paper of the ACR incidental findings committee. Journal of the American College of Radiology, 15(7), pp.966-972.
  - Hoang JK, Langer JE, Middleton WD, Wu CC, Hammers LW, Cronan JJ, Tessler FN, Grant EG, Berland LL. **Managing incidental thyroid nodules detected on imaging: white paper of the ACR Incidental Thyroid Findings Committee.** Journal of the American College of Radiology. 2015 Feb 1;12(2):143-50.

- Head and Neck Cancer:
  - Glastonbury CM, Mukherji SK, O'Sullivan B, Lydiatt WM. **Setting the stage for 2018: how the changes in the American joint committee on cancer/Union for International Cancer Control cancer staging manual eighth edition impact radiologists.** American Journal of Neuroradiology. 2017 Dec 1;38(12):2231-7.

- Brachial Plexus:
  - Tharin BD, Kini JA, York GE, Ritter JL. **Brachial plexopathy: a review of traumatic and nontraumatic causes**. American Journal of Roentgenology. 2014 Jan;202(1):W67-75.
  - Gilcrease-Garcia BM, Deshmukh SD, Parsons MS. **Anatomy, imaging, and pathologic conditions of the brachial plexus.** RadioGraphics. 2020 Oct;40(6):1686-714.

- Lumbar Plexus:
  - Neufeld EA, Shen PY, Nidecker AE, Runner G, Bateni C, Tse G, Chin C. **MR imaging of the lumbosacral plexus: a review of techniques and pathologies.** Journal of Neuroimaging. 2015 Sep;25(5):691-703.
  - Allen H, et al. **MRI of the Lumbosacral Plexus: What the Practicing Radiologist Needs to Know.** https://skeletalrad.org/sites/default/files/pdf/23%20-%20MRI%20of%20the%20Lumbosacral%20Plexus-%20What%20the%20Practicing%20Radiologist%20Needs%20to%20Know.pdf Accessed: 4/26/2021

  - Soldatos T, Andreisek G, Thawait GK, Guggenberger R, Williams EH, Carrino JA, Chhabra A. **High-resolution 3-T MR neurography of the lumbosacral plexus.** Radiographics. 2013 Jul;33(4):967-87.

- Vessel Wall Imaging:
  - Young CC, Bonow RH, Barros G, Mossa-Basha M, Kim LJ, Levitt MR. **Magnetic resonance vessel wall imaging in cerebrovascular diseases. Neurosurgical focus.** 2019 Dec 1;47(6):E4.
  - Lindenholz A, van der Kolk AG, Zwanenburg JJ, Hendrikse J. **The use and pitfalls of intracranial vessel wall imaging: how we do it.** Radiology. 2018 Jan;286(1):12-28.

- MR Spectroscopy:
  - Sitter B, Sjøbakk TE, Larsson HB, Kvistad KA. **Clinical MR spectroscopy of the brain.** Tidsskrift for den Norske laegeforening: tidsskrift for praktisk medicin, ny raekke. 2019 Mar 25;139(6).
  - Öz G, Alger JR, Barker PB, Bartha R, Bizzi A, Boesch C, Bolan PJ, Brindle KM, Cudalbu C, Dinçer A, Dydak U. **Clinical proton MR spectroscopy in central nervous system disorders.** Radiology. 2014 Mar;270(3):658-79.

- MR Perfusion for Tumor:
  - Essig M, Nguyen TB, Shiroishi MS, Saake M, Provenzale JM, Enterline DS, Anzalone N, Dörfler A, Rovira À, Wintermark M, Law M. **Perfusion MRI: the five most frequently asked clinical questions.** American Journal of Roentgenology. 2013 Sep;201(3):W495-510.
  - Griffith B, Jain R. **Perfusion imaging in neuro-oncology: basic techniques and clinical applications.** Radiologic Clinics of North America. 2015 May 1;53(3):497-511.Neska-Matuszewska M, Bladowska J, Sąsiadek M, Zimny A.

- fMRI:
    - Silva MA, See AP, Essayed WI, Golby AJ, Tie Y. **Challenges and techniques for presurgical brain mapping with functional MRI.** NeuroImage: Clinical. 2018 Jan 1;17:794-803.

- Procedures:
    - Hudgins PA, Fountain AJ, Chapman PR, Shah LM. **Difficult lumbar puncture: pitfalls and tips from the trenches.** American Journal of Neuroradiology. 2017 Jul 1;38(7):1276-83.
    - Patel DM, Weinberg BD, Hoch MJ. **CT myelography: clinical indications and imaging findings.** Radiographics. 2020 Mar;40(2):470-84.

- 4D CT for parathyroid Adenomas:
    - Hoang JK, Sung WK, Bahl M, Phillips CD. **How to perform parathyroid 4D CT: tips and traps for technique and interpretation.** Radiology. 2014 Jan;270(1):15-24.

- Fetal MRI:
    - Saleem SN. **Fetal MRI: An approach to practice: A review.** Journal of advanced research. 2014 Sep 1;5(5):507-23.
    - Masselli G, Notte MV, Zacharzewska-Gondek A, Laghi F, Manganaro L, Brunelli R. **Fetal MRI of CNS abnormalities.** Clinical radiology. 2020 Apr 26.

Additional Curated Review Articles

The following are other favorite reviews covering various topics across neuroradiology. These could be referred to as needed or up to interest.

- Surgical Planning:
    - O'Brien Sr WT, Hamelin S, Weitzel EK. **The preoperative sinus CT: avoiding a "CLOSE" call with surgical complications.** Radiology. 2016 Oct;281(1):10-21.
    - Patel PK et al. **"Orthognathic Surgery."** Emedicine. https://emedicine.medscape.com/article/1279747-overview#showall. Accessed: 4/15/2020.

- Special Types of Ischemia:
    - Zalewski NL, Rabinstein AA, Krecke KN, Brown RD, Wijdicks EF, Weinshenker BG, Kaufmann TJ, Morris JM, Aksamit AJ, Bartleson JD, Lanzino G. **Characteristics of spontaneous spinal cord infarction and proposed diagnostic criteria.** JAMA neurology. 2019 Jan 1;76(1):56-63.
    - Huang, Benjamin Y., and Mauricio Castillo. **"Hypoxic-ischemic brain injury: imaging findings from birth to adulthood."** Radiographics 28.2 (2008): 417-439.

- Seizures:
    - Cianfoni A, Caulo M, Cerase A, Della Marca G, Falcone C, Di Lella GM, Gaudino S, Edwards J, Colosimo C. **Seizure-induced brain lesions: a wide spectrum of variably reversible MRI abnormalities.** European journal of radiology. 2013 Nov 1;82(11):1964-72.

- Perineural Tumor Spread:
    - Maroldi R, Farina D, Borghesi A, Marconi A, Gatti E. **Perineural tumor spread.** Neuroimaging clinics of North America. 2008 May 1;18(2):413-29.'

- Spine Imaging:
  - Kotsenas AL. **Imaging of posterior element axial pain generators: facet joints, pedicles, spinous processes, sacroiliac joints, and transitional segments.** Radiologic Clinics. 2012 Jul 1;50(4):705-30.
  - Fardon DF, Williams AL, Dohring EJ, Murtagh FR, Rothman SL, Sze GK. **Lumbar disc nomenclature: version 2.0: Recommendations of the combined task forces of the North American Spine Society, the American Society of Spine Radiology and the American Society of Neuroradiology.** The Spine Journal. 2014 Nov 1;14(11):2525-45.

- Uncommon Infection:
  - Razek AA, Watcharakorn A, Castillo M. **Parasitic diseases of the central nervous system.** Neuroimaging Clinics. 2011 Nov 1;21(4):815-41.

- Dementia:
  - Patel KP, Wymer DT, Bhatia VK, Duara R, Rajadhyaksha CD. **Multimodality imaging of dementia: Clinical importance and role of integrated anatomic and molecular imaging.** RadioGraphics. 2020 Jan;40(1):200-22.

- Teeth:
  - Dean, K. E. "**A Radiologist's Guide to Teeth: An Imaging Review of Dental Anatomy, Nomenclature, Trauma, Infection, and Tumors.**" Neurographics 10.5-6 (2020): 302-318.

- COVID:
  - Chougar L, Shor N, Weiss N, Galanaud D, Leclercq D, Mathon B, Belkacem S, Stroër S, Burrel S, Boutolleau D, Demoule A. **Retrospective observational study of brain magnetic resonance imaging findings in patients with acute SARS-CoV-2 infection and neurological manifestations.** Radiology. 2020 Jul 17.

- Fraser, J.F., Arthur, A.S., Chen, M., Levitt, M., Mocco, J., Albuquerque, F.C., Ansari, S.A., Dabus, G., Jayaraman, M.V., Mack, W.J. and Milburn, J., 2020. **Society of NeuroInterventional Surgery recommendations for the care of emergent neurointerventional patients in the setting of COVID-19.** Journal of neurointerventional surgery, 12(6), pp.539-541.

Last Thoughts on Approach

You may note that some fellows may get by with doing a less structured/curriculum-driven approach. A case-based curriculum, e.g., looking up entities and exam types and doing review articles, can be very useful.

That being said, use some degree of top-down approach is recommended, particularly at the beginning of fellowship. This helps deal with the issue of "not knowing what you don't know" and includes making sure you're at least familiar with uncommon/rare high-risk entities. A comprehensive approach can be particularly helpful also if you're going to be a referral center and seeing a larger number of complex or difficult cases.

Doing any significant proportion of the above should be enough to prepare you for the subspecialty part of the certifying exam (e.g., 3 neuroradiology sections) and CAQ. If you're interested in more information, these topics have been well written about by Brent Weinberg and Ben White here:

- https://learnneuroradiology.com/examprep/neuro-caq/
- https://learnneuroradiology.com/examprep/abr-certifying-exam/
- https://www.benwhite.com/radiology/the-abr-certifying-exam/

I'd also like to highly recommend their writing on neuroradiology, medicine, and other topics. There are excellent resource recommendations and teaching videos contained in their respective websites as well.

Dictation Efficiency and Macros

Long H. Tu

Mehmet Emin Adin

Balaji Rao

Introduction

The following applies perhaps to all of radiology. Even though with time, you'll get faster and more efficient at looking at the studies, there is a limit to how fast it's possible to actually look without sacrificing thoroughness and accuracy.

Therefore, the remaining modifiable factor to improve speed is to maximize dictation efficiency. When you're required to move fast, the goal should be to minimize the number of words you have to say on any given report, while still commenting on all findings that have clinical relevance or that will change management. I should emphasize that these are strategies for use when you're under enough constraint that patient care would suffer if you do not maximize reporting speed. Your search and analysis of the images and medical data should remain 100% thorough, but you can optimize the efficiency of communicating those findings.

Dictate to Guide Management, Not to Enumerate Abnormality

A good place to start is to consider what alteration in care will result from your report and work backwards.

- Ask yourself:
    - What is the change in management that will likely occur as a result of this study?
    - What is the fewest number of words I can use in the impression to motivate the expected change in management?
    - What the least amount of text I can put in the findings to justify the impression?
    - What is the least amount of talking to the dictaphone I can do that allows me to compose the report that satisfies the above conditions?
    - What library of macros/templates should I have at the ready, that I can speak as little as possible to describe common findings, so that I can focus on the high-level work?

- A few strategies arise from this orientation.
  - For exams where there is no change, or that are basically normal, consider writing impressions such as:
    - "Stable exam."
    - "Negative MRI"
  - For stable/negative exams with inconsequential incidental findings or changes unlikely to alter management, consider:
    - "No evidence of acute process."
    - "No acute abnormality."
  - In the findings section, if you're pressed for time, consider wording such as:
    - "No other significant change from prior."
    - "Stable chronic/incidental findings."

- Consider using as few words as absolutely required to describe the features and changes in findings, when you have to mention them at all.
  - Consider using noun-phrases rather than full sentences.
    - Instead of: "There is stable T2/FLAIR hyperintensity surrounding the lesion."
    - Consider: "Stable perilesional T2/FLAIR hyperintensity."
  - A lot of wording commonly used in radiology reporting is unnecessary and adds no information. If a finding is stable or most likely inconsequential, describe as briefly as possible. Findings where there is a very short differential, or where there underlying entity is known or near 100% likely, could be named rather than described.
    - Instead of: "There is an extra-axial, homogeneously enhancing mass at the right frontal convexity previously characterized as a meningioma. It measures 0.3 x 0.4 x 0.5 cm (AP x TV x CC), previously 0.2 x 0.4 x 0.4 cm on MRI performed 7 years prior. There is contact of the underlying brain parenchyma without parenchymal signal abnormality or mass effect."
    - Consider: "Minimally larger, 0.5 cm right frontal meningioma. No mass effect."

- You can also group stable/non-contributory findings together, describing with broad strokes.
  - Instead of… "There is hypodensity and volume loss at the right frontal lobe, right parietal lobe, and left cerebellum, unchanged from prior. There are lacunar infarcts at the right thalamus, right putamen, and left pons. These are unchanged from prior. There are scattered hypodensities in the periventricular and subcortical white matter, which are non-specific, though could represent sequela of small vessel ischemia. These are similar compared to prior"
  - Consider (if none would change management): "Stable multifocal encephalomalacia, lacunar infarcts, and white matter changes."

Maximize Macro-Based Efficiency

- Use macros (or pick-lists) as much as possible to minimize unnecessary/redundant dictation.
  - The following are a few categories of findings that you can avoid dictating in full because of how common they are (use a macro instead!)
    - White matter changes.
    - Volume loss.
    - Lacunar infarcts.
    - No spinal stenosis.
    - Etc.

- Consider substituting the normal lines in your templates with pick lists for the most common abnormalities (such as above). This can make you even more efficient, as then you don't even need to call the macro verbally.
  - For example, include a line in your MRI brain template that reads "[No confluent parenchymal signal abnormality.]" This can be used as the default option a series of pick-able choices including differing degrees of white matter disease.

    - [*Scattered* hypodensities in the periventricular and subcortical white matter are non-specific, though could represent sequela of chronic small vessel ischemia.]
    - [*Scattered* and *patchy* hypodensities in the periventricular and subcortical white matter are non-specific, though could represent sequela of chronic small vessel ischemia.]
    - [*Extensive patchy and confluent* hypodensities in the periventricular and subcortical white matter are non-specific, though could represent sequela of chronic small vessel ischemia.]
  - Using such a strategy can make you even more efficient by making it so that you don't have to even dictate a command/macro to populate common findings.
  - Another example: consider pick-lists for sometimes tiresome-to-describe degenerative changes. For example, my own lumbar spine template has a line that reads: "At L5-S1, there is [no significant disc abnormality]."
  - The bracketed phrase can be replaced via pick-list with:
    - [a broad-based disc bulge]
    - [a broad-based disc bulge and facet arthropathy]
    - [a broad-based disc bulge, facet arthropathy, and thickening of the ligamentum flavum]
    - [a broad-based disc bulge, facet arthropathy, and thickening of the ligamentum flavum]
    - [a broad-based disc bulge, facet arthropathy, thickening of the ligamentum flavum, and prominent epidural fat]
  - The subsequent lines reads: "This produces [no significant] spinal canal stenosis, [no significant] right neuroforaminal stenosis, and [no significant] left neuroforaminal stenosis."

- Each of the above bracketed items can then be replaced via pick list with
    - [mild]
    - [moderate]
    - [severe]
- Note that much of what we describe in degenerative change, outside of severe pathology has little correlation with patient symptoms or presentation. If what you're describing will ultimately do nothing for the patient, consider using these sorts of mechanisms to move quickly. If you're describing likely symptomatic or clinically significant changes, it can be worthwhile to go into more detail.
- Building (or obtaining, see end of chapter) templates such as these early in training can make you a lot faster and allow you to focus on higher level work.

- Instead of frequently modifying the pre-populated macro to describe incidental findings of no consequence, consider changing your default macro so that you only ever *have* to modify it if there are important findings. Therefore, if you forget or do not want to add small details, the statements remain technically correct. For example:
    - Instead of modifying a default statement such as "The orbits are unremarkable" to "Status post bilateral lens replacements." (Which usually does not alter management) … Change your default macro to "No acute orbital pathology."
    - Instead of modifying "The paranasal sinuses are clear" every time you see a polyp/mucous retention cyst or minimal secretions… Change your default macro to read "There is no significant mucosal thickening in the paranasal sinuses."
        - Note that some literature suggests that mucosal thickening ≤3mm is probably physiologic/of no consequence. You probably don't need to comment.
        - See: *Rak KM, Newell 2nd JD, Yakes WF, Damiano MA, Luethke JM. Paranasal sinuses on MR images of the brain: significance of mucosal thickening. AJR. American journal of roentgenology. 1991 Feb;156(2):381-4.*

  - Instead of modifying "The ventricles and sulci are normal in size" every time you see parenchymal volume loss or ex vacuo dilatation… Change you default macro to "No evidence of acute hydrocephalus."
  - The above principle can be applied to every anatomic section where you find yourself noting findings that are incidental and do not change management, just because the finding makes your template technically false. "[Anatomy]: [No acute finding.]" is a nice formula if applicable to your institutional practice.

- Note that the format of your macros plays a large role in report readability and ease of editing.
  - Consider using bullet points for findings in your templates, rather than having them all run together in one paragraph. This can make it much easier to find what you need to modify when dictating.
  - Consider putting a space between each series of bullet points corresponding to a large anatomic compartment such as for intracranial, extra-axial and extracranial anatomy. This can make it even easier to find what you need to change.
  - Organized templates make it easier for clinicians and other radiologists to read your report. It also makes it easier for you to find what you're looking for when you read follow ups for your own studies.

- Consider reading the excellent first reference at the end of the chapter, which elaborates on many of the above concepts.

Prioritize Safety and Continuous Improvement Over Perfection

- To avoid "perseverating" on studies, develop consistent search patterns, and accept that you'll miss things. When you miss something, modify your search pattern rather than developing a habit of looking over every study a needless number of extra times hoping you'll catch additional findings.

- Incorporate your blind spots into default macros so that you're both reminded, and don't need to specifically dictate extra words to reassure yourself that you looked.
- As a trainee, you're not expected to know or see everything. You will miss things. It is important to focus more on continuing to improve, rather than perfection. Seeing and learning from more cases, especially at the beginning of the year, is more useful than approaching every study with the intention of 100% guaranteeing that you'll catch every subtle finding prior to attending review (this is impossible anyways).
- While it is important to aim to detect all potentially impactful findings, the most important thing is to detect all "do-not-miss" lesions and to answer the clinical question. Speed and prioritizing high risk findings are most relevant for call or other high acuity situations. Moving toward a more completionism orientation is more relevant as the year goes on, and you approach full independence.
- Therefore, for any given study, if you've gone through your full search pattern, looked closely at common blinds pots, and checked for high-risk pathology, you can be confident that you've done due diligence.
- You'll keep missing things as an attending, so expect it to continue happening. Try to avoid the worst errors, and use each miss as an opportunity for growth.

Shared Macro Library Link

- Learn from (and steal!) efficiency and reference-oriented macros here: https://tinyurl.com/neurorad-macros.

References:

1. Hartung MP, Bickle IC, Gaillard F, Kanne JP. How to Create a Great Radiology Report. RadioGraphics. 2020 Oct;40(6):1658-70.
2. Eberhardt SC, Heilbrun ME. Radiology report value equation. Radiographics. 2018 Oct;38(6):1888-96.

Common Errors on Neuroimaging Studies

Long H. Tu

Sandra Abi Fadel

Anthony Abou Karam

Introduction

The purpose of this section is to give you a "heads up" as to where fellows tend to miss the most findings and where they make errors in workflow management or interpretation. At the fellowship level, you're likely to have already built search patterns for most exam types, so I won't go into that process in detail, but rather just highlight the most missed findings for common exams and provide some tips on how to avoid them. This section reflects a synthesis of the existing literature as well as surveys of attending neuroradiologists and co-fellows.

Please note that only exams that trainees are expected to have familiarity with from residency are covered in this chapter. Uncommon and advanced studies (MRI of the lumbar plexus, fetal MRI, fMRI, etc.) are discussed in dedicated sections later in the text.

General Workflow and Habits

Fellowship is a time to hone not just knowledge, but the habits that will allow you to practice at a high level consistently. Below are common errors applicable to almost all study types.

- Failure to review the medical chart.
    - The provided indication is frequently wrong or incomplete. Depending on the scenario, clinicians will use a dropdown menu item to fill this field, which does not correspond with the reason they want the study.
    - Even seemingly routine indications can be misleading. For example, "multiple sclerosis – follow up" will be provided, when the actual diagnosis is in question, and any number of infectious/inflammatory or neoplastic entities are still in the differential from a clinical perspective. Do not fall into these sorts of traps.
    - Chart review will change your dictation and how it affects patient care more frequently than many other routine efforts in radiology/medicine. This is especially true for outside (second) interpretation exams, where the reason for a second read and crucial patient history can be buried in scanned documents or other less obvious locations.
    - Documentation of at least some chart review in the study dictation can help assure your attending staff (and subsequently referring providers) that you're invested in due diligence/consulting in the context of the patient as a whole, rather than just report imaging findings.
    - Wherever you end up practicing, there will be pressure to interpret and dictate studies quickly. It is essential to build the habit of reviewing the patient chart early on. Sometimes you may leave a bit later as a result of doing a thorough job. However, in the long run, this can save you time by helping you avoid errors, patient harm, and potentially litigation.
    - Bottom line: never trust the provided indication. Expect it to be misleading every time, and you'll be right frequently. Document generously.

- Not comparing across multiple priors for studies with short-interval follow up (especially for tumor/metastatic disease follow ups), when necessary.
    - Subtle changes in brain lesions, whether primary tumors, metastases, or vascular/developmental processes can be easily missed if the patient is followed on a monthly basis or some other frequent interval.
    - Using 3D co-registration/overlay, if your PACS allows it, can sometimes help with detection of very subtle new abnormalities. Looking at any first presentation or pre-treatment oncologic imaging for example, can give you a sense of the likely appearance of recurrent disease. While the pattern of enhancement or signal abnormality may not be exactly the same (or consistent), this can help in some tricky scenarios. Knowing exactly where original lesion is can also help prime you to locations with higher chance of recurrence.
    - For example, knowing that a primary brain tumor has T2/FLAIR hyperintensity without enhancement, will prime you to look for *specifically* for subtle T2/FLAIR abnormality in follow ups, and not rely on post-contrast images. Just because a lesion does not enhance does not mean that this is not new/progressive disease.
    - Low grade tumors (e.g., oligodendroglioma) may look very similar to the most recent study. Look at follow up studies back at least 2-3 years, especially for follow up of primary brain neoplasms.

- Neglecting prior studies of differing modalities.
    - It's obvious to compare to the most recent MRI for MRI studies, same with CT. However, in some cases, prior nuclear medicine studies, PET/CTs, radiographs and others can hold important information. It's a good rule of thumb to at least check the most recent study of *all* modalities that images the same anatomy as you're looking at currently.
    - Here's an odd example: if you can't tell if a cervical spine compression fracture is chronic, and the patient has no prior CT/MRI/XR of the cervical spine, you can every once in a

while, see the same anatomy on an old fluoroscopic swallow study. This has worked more than once!
    - Another point: intraprocedural (surgical/biopsy) images, prior angiograms, incidental imaging at the edges of studies for other anatomy – these can be useful if you're having a hard time finding a good comparison.

- Not looking very closely at all the localizer images.
    - It can be extremely dangerous to gloss over the localizer images for any exam. If you read enough studies, you *will* see incidental cancers and other high-risk pathology. Treat every localizer image as a legitimate part of the study itself, and go carefully and meticulously through every single part of each of these. Pay special attention to anatomy that is not seen on the conventional sequences.
    - For example, in the lumbar spine, you'll see tumors in the liver, spleen, visceral pelvis, osseous pelvis, and femurs. Coronal localizers for cervical spine MRIs can show you apical lung masses.
    - Total spine MRIs often image nearly the whole body, so you can see brain parenchymal/skull base lesions and basically any visceral disease.
    - Treat every localizer as an incidental additional MRI study, where you'll need to do a quick search pattern through all the anatomy. With this perspective, you'll be better protected from missing serious pathology.
    - Some institutions will do whole-spine localizers to allow "gold standard" numbering of the vertebra from the C1-C2 level. We have seen (and missed) masses of the cauda equina on whole spine localizers of the cervical spine, skull base pathology on localizers for the lumbar spine, etc.

- Not routinely windowing MRI sequences.
    - Frequently, the default windowing of MRI sequences is not advantageous for the detection of subtle lesions. It is a good habit to re-window and level most/all sequences, especially as you look for pathology in differing compartments of the same image set.

- The image invert function can also be useful to detect subtle signal/architectural abnormalities. This can make small strokes more visible on DWI and subtle brain edema more visible on T2/FLAIR. Cortical malformations can be more visible with image inversion as well.
- Windowing is particularly helpful when looking for strokes in the posterior fossa. Find a balance between susceptibility/artifact at the skull base and true restricted diffusion. You may need differing windows for the supratentorial and infratentorial brain.
- Note that if you obtain both axial and coronal DWI/ADC images, that you might see a small stroke on only one reconstruction. Do not dismiss a finding just because you don't see it on the other acquisition! Thick slabs in either direction can miss small abnormality.

- Errors of cognitive bias: expecting stable/negative/unremarkable.
    - If you're reading a study where the provided indication orscenario seems not entirely appropriate or where there's a couple of recent priors have been stable/negative, this creates an expectation that the study will not find something new, even before you start looking. This is one of the most dangerous scenarios, and you should recognize it as such.
    - This sort of bias also applies when studies are technically limited. It can be easy to slip into the thinking of "oh, I won't be able to see anything, so this will just be non-diagnostic." You can still very often find real pathology on even nearly-nondiagnostic studies.
    - If you go into looking at a study with the expectation that it will not yield a new or concerning finding, you will miss critical pathology. Many radiologists (myself included!), have passed strokes, subtle bleeds, and cancers, or have continued to re-state incorrect diagnoses under the sway of expecting something to be stable/negative.
    - This bias is extremely difficult to overcome. One of the few ways to combat this is to go into every study with the *expectation* that you'll find something unexpected and subtle.

You will only see what you expect to find, so if you're looking for subtlety, you will do better at detecting it.

- Resist the cynicism that can arise from ordering patterns (by provider/clinical service/location) that seem low value or "inappropriate" at first glance. It is extremely dangerous to suspect a study will be negative before you open it. If you're encountering frustration with low value use, please consider addressing this at the workflow, policy, and research/QI level. Separate this impulse from the demands of any given study that arises in your clinical responsibility.
- For any given study (and indication/scenario), it can be useful to ask yourself "what do I definitely not want to miss?" and make you double-check for subtle findings along these lines – especially if you can sense yourself becoming less engaged.
- When repeated studies are done for a specific indication (e.g., MRAs for aneurysm, MRI for multiple sclerosis, etc.), it is *very* easy to fall into the trap of only looking for change in the obvious or known abnormality. We have seen/missed strokes on DWI images on one of many MRAs for aneurysm follow up. New parotid masses have been seen/missed on routine follow up MRIs for MS plaques.
- Don't just look for the things a clinician could also easily find. Look for the things that a clinician would miss (would not even know to look for), if they were to open the study.

- Failure to proofread.
  - Obviously, be most attentive to the impression, and sections of writing that directly impact care.
  - With patients increasingly able to access their own medical charts and reports, even seemingly inconsequential dictation errors will come under scrutiny. Patients can (and will) read every line and every word of their own reports.

- Failure to maximize learning from mistakes.
  - Always review all final reports for changes and missed findings.
  - Read about anything where errors reveal gaps in knowledge.

- If you notice a pattern of misses (which can be specific to each person), make sure to modify your search pattern. Better yet, modify your templates to include reminders. For example, my CTA head and neck template includes wording that directs me to check both the venous sinuses and incidentally imaged pulmonary arteries on every case. This is a reaction to missing thrombi at these sites in the past.

Non-Contrast CT Head

I include this bread-and-butter exam because it is so common that driving down error rates here would have a disproportionate impact on overall error rates.

- Missing subtle blood:
    - Most common sites of subtle, missed hemorrhage: along the falx and tentorium, dependently within the occipital horns of the lateral ventricles, sulci at the vertex, posterior 3rd ventricle, at the interpeduncular cistern, inferior aspect of brain/foramen magnum. Near-isodense blood is particularly easy to miss.
    - Scroll more slowly, with tight windowing, thin cuts, and multiple projections through danger zones above. Enumerate the expected CSF spaces mentally as you search through them.
    - When you find a subdural (or other blood) on one side in the setting of trauma, look *very* carefully on the other side, as you'll very frequently find another subtle abnormality.
    - It's best to use not just thin axials, but also thin coronal reconstructions.

- Missing subtle strokes:
    - Most common sites of subtle, missed strokes: occipital lobe, posterior fossa, and new small lacunar infarcts. Small strokes at the cortex near the vertex (first few axial images) are also very easy to miss.
    - Use tightly windowed, thick-slab reconstructions. Also look in coronal and sagittal reconstructions for stroke (not just axials!). Look through the ACA/PCA and vertebrobasilar territories every exam! It can be useful to start by looking at these, and save the more common/obvious MCA territory for last in your search pattern.
    - Don't forget to look at the venous anatomy consistently for hyperdensity, i.e., venous thrombosis. Not all stroke is arterial in etiology.

  - Chronic small vessel disease (multiple areas of hypodensity), can confuse the picture, and make it very difficult to detect new ischemia. It's essential to compare to priors, ideally with co-registration. If there are no priors, or it is unclear whether hypodensities are new, consider MRI. We have seen extensive multifocal infarcts be nearly invisible on CT in this setting.

- Other common misses:
  - It's extremely easy to miss mass lesions in the upper neck/face at the edge of the study. Don't forget to include these in your search pattern for every study. Always check the nasopharynx (especially if there's a mastoid effusion).
  - Especially in oncologic patients, look for preservation of the skull base foramina. New perineural disease can be subtle and easily missed when these patients are imaged for concern of "acute intracranial process."
  - Abnormalities of the orbits and calvarium can be easy to pass over if the provided indication does not direct your attention. Make sure to check the superior ophthalmic veins on every study (clue to intracranial vascular pathology). Make sure to differentiate suspicious calvarial lucencies from venous lakes, hemangiomas, and other common reasons for heterogeneous appearance of the bone.

CT Neck Notes

Much of CT neck imaging done at the fellowship level is for head and neck cancer. This is a large topic which cannot be covered completely here. However, to get you started, it's useful to provide a few pointers and direction for deeper reading as needed. In short, head and neck cancer staging has recently changed (2018). The criteria are different from many other cancers in the body, so you cannot just port what you know from other cancers. For example, head and neck lymph nodes should be measured in *largest* dimension, in contrast to most sites. Depending on P16 status, you'll have to discuss potential extranodal extension of disease (ENE).

For *any* caner you evaluate, whether in the head and neck or elsewhere, it is good practice to have the most recent AJCC staging guide open real time. This can help you understand what features you have to comment on for any given malignancy. Below are a few essential considerations applicable to the CT neck imaging for malignancy. A brief set of common errors and misses for all CT neck imaging is provided afterward.

- Checklist for head and neck malignancies:
  - Protocol oral cavity/mucosal tumors to be performed with a "puffed" cheek technique.
  - Always have the recent AJCC staging information open for cancer studies (unless you know it well).
  - Review the chart to know if the patient is P16+ or P16-. This is marker for HPV infection. If you don't know or can't find the in formation, presume the patient is P16-.
    - For P16- cancers, you'll have to specifically report any extranodal extension of disease.
    - Extranodal extension of disease is suggested by indistinct nodal margins, irregular nodal capsular enhancement, or infiltration into adjacent structures.
  - Measure/report all lymph nodes in long axis.
  - Note whether nodes are conglomerate or not.
  - Look carefully for osseus involvement.
  - An easy blind spot is retropharyngeal lymph nodes, both medial and lateral. Look specifically for these, and comment on presence, enlargement, and/or abnormal morphology.

    - Make sure you check all the fat planes in the neck. Remember to look for perineural spread of tumor. Look for muscle atrophy.
    - When you see a tumor, comment on whether or not it encases the carotid arteries.
- Common errors/blind spots on all head and neck imaging.
    - Retromolar trigone – make sure you evaluated this area on thin cuts, with multiple planes. This is especially important if there are abnormal nodes, and you cannot find the primary lesion.
    - Parathyroid glands and masses are easy to dismiss as part of thyroid. Be care to distinguish from exophytic nodules by enhancement/attenuation and any subtle fat planes.
    - Do not forget to check the lung apices and mediastinum. Synchronous/metachronous lung cancers or metastatic disease is often missed on CT neck imaging.
    - Don't forget to look at the skull base and spinal canal.

References:

1. Glastonbury CM, Salzman KL. Pitfalls in the staging of cancer of nasopharyngeal carcinoma. Neuroimaging Clinics. 2013 Feb 1;23(1):9-25.
2. Glastonbury CM, Mukherji SK, O'Sullivan B, Lydiatt WM. Setting the stage for 2018: how the changes in the American joint committee on cancer/Union for International Cancer Control cancer staging manual eighth edition impact radiologists. American Journal of Neuroradiology. 2017 Dec 1;38(12):2231-7.

CTA Head and Neck

CTA head and neck use is rising, partly related to selection of patients for thrombectomy in acute ischemic stroke. This has become the de facto imaging exam for any patient with potentially neurovascular pathology, which covers a large variety of clinical scenarios.

In some instances (at our institution) the non-contrast CT head and CTA head and neck portions are reported separately, by differing radiologists. This is done to expedite reporting, especially of the non-contrast CT, to exclude hemorrhage. When these studies are reported separately, it's useful to still correlate with the concurrent exam, as you may see something in the larger context that explains or makes it easier to detect findings on the study you're reporting.

- Tips on real-time consultation in stroke:
  - At our institution, if there is a "stroke code," we may be consulting real time with the vascular neurology service that is managing the patient. They will often call before/while the study is in progress. This can be flustering if you're managing a slew of acute/hyperacute cases, and there is a tendency to miss the opportunity to provide extremely high-value, timely consultation. The expectation is not to provide a full "wet-read" of the *entire* study… the stroke neurologist needs you to answer only two questions: "Is there blood in the head?" (i.e., a contraindication to tPA) and "Is there a large vessel occlusion (LVO)?".
  - The stroke team will often be with the patient if there is a high probability that the patient has a true ischemic event. They will want to know if there is intracranial hemorrhage. If you will also be reporting an accompanying non-contrast CT head, you can just run the part of your search pattern for intracranial hemorrhage and verbally communicate that quickly. Given the real-time/high-risk nature of this consultation, and depending on the institution, stroke neurologists may also be looking at the exam and assessing for blood. It is ultimately their decision whether or not to give tPA, so if you're not comfortable for any reason, you

can be clear that the verbal communication is preliminary, and that a final interpretation will be following very shortly.

- Be extremely wary of the pitfalls of real-time interpretation. With the pressure of time, someone standing at the workstation with urgent questions, or interrupting you, you will not be able to function at a normal level of accuracy. Once you field directed questions to the best of your ability, it is best to double check parts of the exam you performed in real time with a thorough, normal search pattern. You will frequently find new abnormalities, or management changing alterations compared to what was possible to provide on the spot, outside of a rigorous approach.

- Consider use of coronal and sagittal MIPs to quickly assess the arteries.
  - Scrolling carefully through the head/neck vasculature on thin axial images may not be efficient enough for real-time consultation.
  - A better strategy is to enter an MPR view, and reorient the imaging planes so that the extracranial arterials are laid out on coronal (or sagittal if you'd like) images. Use a combination of medium/thick MIPs and averaged projections to quickly assess the carotid and vertebral system this way. I usually assess the neck vessels on coronals first and use the sagittals as a double check. Axials are only for troubleshooting.
  - Modify the planes as necessary to similarly assess the intracranial vasculature. I find the axials and coronals to most useful for the anterior circulation. Coronals are often the best for posterior circulation, with axials/sagittals as needed. Sagittal MIPS can be useful for assessment of the M3/M4 MCA branches.
  - If consulting real time for concern of LVO, you only need to look at the ICAs, M1 segments (+/- proximal M2s), and the vertebrobasilar system, so this should only take a few seconds. Proximal ACA/PCA is nice to check when there are referrable symptoms. It should be emphasized that the

point is not to find *all* occlusions, but to give quick consultation for potential triage to thrombectomy.
  - Therefore, a useful default script is "There's no LVO. I don't see blood in the head. The final report will be following shortly, and I'll get back to you if there are major discrepancies."

- Most commonly missed findings on the CTA neck portion:
  - It is very easy to pass carotid webs and other small findings on the axial images. As above, use reformatted oblique coronal and sagittals as often as possible. The arterial "beading" of fibromuscular dysplasia can be easily missed on axials, best seen on coronals.
  - Look carefully at not just the carotid/vertebral arteries, but also the arch vessels. It is very easy to pass high grade stenosis at the origin of the subclavian or brachiocephalic arteries. Remember that these can produce steal phenomena. The degree of stenosis is often best characterized on axial images for the arch.
  - It can be very easy to miss incidental findings in the non-vascular anatomy. Make sure to evaluate each part of the anatomy step-by-step. The easiest to miss and highest risk findings are pulmonary embolism, incidental pulmonary nodules, and thoracic adenopathy (supraclavicular, mediastinal, and even axillary). Look through the pulmonary arteries as closely as the contrast bolus timing allows on every CTA head and neck. Make sure you look at the whole neck soft tissues, include the aerodigestive track/mucosal surfaces and nodal distributions.
  - Potentially explanatory findings that are easy to dismiss include high grade spinal stenosis, which can sometimes correlate with neurologic symptoms if there is not a clear vascular etiology.
  - Note that if a CTA head and neck is performed concurrent with a non-contrast CT head exam, it's not just upper chest and neck that you see only on the CTA. The inferior aspects of the maxillary sinuses, nasal cavity, oral cavity, and lower

face/mandible might only be seen on the CTA part of the study. Make sure you look at all these closely.
  - Make sure to look at the bones closely --- you'll see fractures/bone lesions that may not be expected with the provided indication.

- Most commonly missed findings on the CT/CTA head portion:
  - The most common missed vessel cut offs are at the M2 and M3 segments of the MCAs. Be very careful to follow both the superior and inferior division branches specifically.
    - Slow down, and use axial and sagittal reconstructions (+/-MIPS at the distal M2 and M3s).
    - Be aware of variant early bifurcation of the MCA, which can be confusing and simulate a distal M1 cutoff.
  - ACA and PCA cut offs after the first segment can also be extremely easy to miss. In most patients, make sure that you see both ACAs as they course superiorly and posteriorly – following each individually as needed. It can be easy to be fooled into thinking both still fill with contrast by tortuous course of the single remaining ACA.
    - Remember that are variants such as ACA trifurcation (3 vessels), or rarely an azygous ACA (1 vessel). Make sure you track the vessels very carefully or compare with priors. Seeing two ACAs could mean that one of three has been occluded! Seeing only one ACA could be "normal" for some patients.
  - Be sure not to confuse a deep cerebral vein with the more distal PCA branches. Make sure you identify these separately on every study. This is an easy pitfall.
  - Be extremely wary of saying "no vessel cut off" when the patient has a localizing presentation. Look especially careful (with every projection) where the lesion localizes by presentation. Multiple planes help detect subtle/focal stenosis in these cases.

- Always look for aneurysms at the most common areas – MCA bifurcations, A-comm complex, and P-comm origin. Additionally, look at commonly missed areas, such as the carotid terminus and basilar tip. Make sure you're using multiple projections, especially the coronals. MIPs can make the search much faster in most of the anatomy.
- Thin MPRs (rather than MIPs) in multiple planes are helpful to assess the ICAs. Their course through the skull base and the tortuosity of the siphons makes it difficult to use MIPs to detect aneurysms or stenosis. Aneurysms of the carotid siphons are easily missed – look closely on thin MPRs.
- Do not forget to look for distal aneurysms in the setting of trauma, infection, or underlying vasculitis.
- It's important to note that if you find one aneurysm (or if the patient has known aneurysms), that the chances that you'll find additional aneurysms goes up. Look extra carefully for more subtle, small aneurysms in these cases.
- Make sure the blind ended outpouchings are aneurysms and not a branch cutoff. Be wary of this pitfall especially around the ACA origins.
- Consider that if you're imaging for imbalance/dizziness, that middle/inner ear pathology can be explanatory. Look specifically for entities such dehiscent semicircular canals (especially the superior one) or middle ear effusions. You may also occasionally see IAC masses. Note that CT/CTA is at most 40% sensitive for small posterior fossa strokes. Make sure to recommend MRI if there is any more than minimal suspicion.
- Consider that hearing loss can mimic cognitive decline or slow onset altered mental status. Make sure to check if the EACs are obstructed or if there are middle ear effusions.

- Miscellaneous notes/tips:
    - You can use tightly windowed thick MIPs as a "poor man's" CT perfusion map. Look for areas of relative decreased vascularity/attenuation of the brain to spot subtle ischemia.
    - Use of the above technique with post-processed subtraction images can allow you even higher sensitivity.

- If your PACS allows it, 3D co-registering a current and prior CTA head can allow you to detect very subtle new vessel stenoses or cut offs. This can help demonstrate M3 or M4 occlusions if you're lucky enough have a recent prior.
- Depending on your institutional protocol and patient characteristics, note that the venous sinuses may opacify (at least partially) on CTA exams. Especially as many indications for CTA are non-localizing/non-specific, you will occasionally see thrombus, or more commonly, transverse sinus narrowing in the setting of intracranial hypertension. Consider adding the venous sinuses to your usual search pattern, or keep a (appropriately hedged) reminder in your default CTA template.

MRI Brain

MRI brain is a somewhat of a misnomer. It's best to think of this also as an MRI of the whole head and upper neck/face. There is a lot of anatomy to check. It is most common to miss important pathology outside the brain parenchyma, so it is essential to look thoroughly at all the peripheral and surrounding structures.

- Pre-contrast T1 (sagittal and axials):
    - *Always* assess the marrow signal of the calvarium, skull base, visualized face, and upper spine. Marrow replacement/metastases are extremely easy to miss.
    - Always check the midline structures. You should also return to these on post-contrast images to assess enhancement characteristics.
        - Look at the pituitary for lesions and the normal "bright spot."
        - Look for corpus callosal abnormalities (dysgenesis, agenesis, thinning, etc.)
        - Look for pineal region masses/cystic lesions.
        - Look at the craniocervical junction for tonsillar ectopia, e.g., as seen in the Chiari malformations.

- DWI/ADC:
    - Window tightly. Look closely at the calvarium for marrow lesions on high B-value images. You can also see upper head and neck adenopathy on these images (e.g., retropharyngeal and level 2/5 nodes). Be sure to look outside of the brain. It can be a good habit to do this first.
    - DWI will show you more than acute ischemia intracranially. Look at the subarachnoid spaces and ventricles for blood and pus. Do not dismiss intraventricular restricted diffusion, presuming that it always represents choroid plexus xanthogranulomas. It can be good practice to look at the CSF spaces next, before the brain.
    - When looking at the brain, scroll very slowly, and be wary of missing punctate infarcts, especially in the brainstem and posterior fossa, where is it is easy to scroll by small findings.

- If there is concern for small posterior fossa stroke (e.g., dizziness, vertigo, incoordination, ataxia) consider adding thin cut coronal DWI/ADC images through the brainstem as part of the protocol.
- Infarcts may not be always seen on both axial and coronal DWI if sufficiently small relative to slice thickness. Do not dismiss a finding seen on only one sequence - especially if it is potentially explanatory.
- Also keep in mind that not everything that restricts diffusion is stroke, especially if subacute stroke is on the differential. Consider that high grade glioma may often restrict diffusion and can incidentally conform to a vascular territory. We have seen tumors look indistinguishable from subacute stroke. Careful history/chart review and follow up made help clarify. Remember that seizures, acute infection/inflammation, and other entities can restrict diffuse. Be careful of falling prey to premature closure.

- SWI:
  - Don't just look at the brain. Look for abnormal CSF space susceptibility. Subtle SAH and other extra-axial blood is easily missed. Look for subtle dependent blood in the ventricles.
  - Also look along the brainstem and cranial nerves, subtle susceptibility is very easy to pass.
  - Look at the vasculature. You can see thrombus/occlusion in both arteries and veins as a "susceptibility vessel sign."
  - Remember that susceptibility is not always blood. It also be calcium, air, metal, other rare materials. Always check the phase map and/or recent CT.

- FLAIR:
  - Do not forget to look at *everything outside the brain*, including the scalp/soft tissues and marrow.
  - Note the 2D coronal and other projections may capture more anatomy than the axials. Make sure to quickly look at the marrow and soft tissues in the upper neck that is seen on this sequence but not the axials.

- Coronal FLAIR is useful for pachymeningeal thickening and thin extra-axial collections that may not be seen well on axials.
- The hippocampi are also well evaluated on coronal FLAIR.
- Pay special attention to the CSF spaces, where FLAIR is often most sensitive for blood, debris, and small collections.
- Look for abnormal signal in the venous sinuses (need to correlate with other sequences/MRV for slow flow vs thrombus).

- T2:
  - Don't forget to check vessel flow voids. Do this for both arterial and venous structures.
  - For non-contrast exams, T2 may be your only chance to see the vessels well. Look for aneurysms at all the usual branch points and vessel ends. You can save a life this way!
  - Don't forget that absent signal in the venous sinuses does NOT mean they are thrombus-free.
  - Make sure to check the optic nerve sheath complexes in intracranial hypertension.
  - Especially for dizziness/hearing related complaints, remember to evaluate the inner ear structures, for cochlear malformations/abnormalities and dehiscent semicircular canals.

- Post-contrast MPRAGE (3D T1/GRE):
  - Do not forget incidental facial anatomy, the upper neck deep spaces, the nasal/oral cavities, teeth, and upper pharynx.
  - *Always* look at all the arteries and venous structures. It can be extremely easy to go by aneurysms or small/peripheral (e.g., sigmoid sinus) thrombi.
  - At the same time, do not assume a venous sinus is patent just because it "fills" homogenously with contrast. Some chronic thrombi may have enhancement. If that is concern for thrombus, make sure to correlate with any phase contrast, TOF, and/or dynamic post-contrast MRV.

- The falx and tentorium are common blind spots. Coronal reformats are particularly useful to look for mass lesions and other abnormalities near these structures.
- You can see the upper cervical arteries on the MPRAGE. This is an opportunity to detect FMD, pseudoaneurysms, etc.
- On sagittal images, sure you take a second look at the pituitary, as you'll see adenomas, cysts, etc.

- Post-contrast spin echo:
  - Do not forget to window these tightly and look as closely as on the MPRAGE/3D T1. These are technically distinct, and obtained at a differing (more delayed) time point.
  - You'll frequently see enhancing lesions (e.g., ventriculitis, cranial nerve enhancement, leptomeningeal, inflammatory) much better. Some late-enhancing lesions may ONLY be seen on the spin echo sequence.
  - If these are VERY delayed (i.e., concurrently imaging total spine) even cysts/abscess may begin filling with contrast.

References:

1. Bahrami S, Yim CM. Quality initiatives: blind spots at brain imaging. Radiographics. 2009 Nov;29(7):1877-96.

CT/MRI Orbits Notes

Orbital lesions can be very subtle. The following applies mostly to dedicated to MRI exams of the orbits, though similar concerns can be applied to CT and the orbital anatomy on MRI brain, face, etc.

- Patients will often receive imaging of the orbits to evaluate an abnormality with vision. Don't forget: underlying lesions can be anywhere from the globe to the visual cortex, inclusive of the retina, optic nerve, chiasm, optic tracks, optic radiations in the white matter, and occipital lobe. Various neurodegenerative processes and other brain lesions may also present with visual abnormalities.

- If there is any possibility that there's a central cause for vision loss, consider protocolling for a concurrent MRI brain. If you are imaging only the orbits, the lesion can either missed or be seen only at the corner or edge of a sequence (e.g., occipital lobe incidentally seen on with FOV centered on orbits).

- Look very carefully for asymmetric T2 signal in the optics nerves on coronal images. If you do not specifically compare the optic nerves on *each* image, you will miss subtle signal abnormality (e.g., optic neuritis). Asymmetric/abnormal signal can be seen posterior to the optic apex, at the chiasm, and sometimes within the optic tracks.

- Inflammatory/infectious processes at the orbital apex can be similarly very subtle. Compare the fat signal and enhancement of each side careful on each image. Window tightly.

- Do not forget to look at the tentorium for subtle thickening if the patient has pain. This can be the earliest sign of Tolosa-Hunt/pseudotumor – easily missed if not looking specifically.

MRI Spine Studies

I'm writing this section as if for an MRI of the total spine. Take any relevant pieces to apply to just a study of just the cervical/thoracic/lumbar anatomy.

- Localizers.
  - It's probably best to approach the MRI total spine like an incidental MRI of the whole body. This can be a difficult concept to embrace if you're attached to the idea of being only a neuroimager. In truth however, the number of significant findings that you find outside the spine can be nearly as many as inside the spine. Symptoms that prompt spine imaging are often so difficult to localize that you'll frequently find explanatory or at least potentially significant findings in the paraspinal/extra-spinal anatomy.
  - Look at the brain, head, neck, chest, abdomen, pelvis, bones, and soft tissues in a systematic, careful pattern for every exam. You will find *a lot* of pathology.
  - Examples of things we've seen missed, or have missed ourselves:
    - In the cervical spine: internal auditory canal mass, cervical adenopathy, thyroid nodes/masses, lung apical masses, jugular vein thrombosis.
    - In the thoracic spine: pulmonary embolus, lung nodules/masses, thoracic adenopathy.
    - In the lumbar spine: adrenal masses, pelvic cystic structures and masses, retroperitoneal nodes, unknown colon cancer.
  - In short – *always* look carefully outside the spine.

- STIR/T2 FS.
  - Don't just look for vertebra body/disc edema. Look at the facets, all the ligaments, skull base, and immediately adjacent soft tissues. Injuries and other explanatory pathology are frequently in these other compartments.
  - Look for fluid in the prevertebral space, which can indicate infection or acute trauma.

    - When you see ONE compression fracture, make sure you look VERY carefully at other levels, where you'll often see very subtle other fractures/marrow edema.
    - If there is an acute fracture, presume that there is ligamentous injury until proven otherwise, and look for it.

- T2/T1 pre-contrast.
    - Do not forget the skull base and imaged brain! You'll frequently see the sella, paranasal sinuses, brainstem, fourth ventricle, and cerebellum on cervical spine imaging. Sellar masses are extremely easy to miss. Posterior fossa masses can also easily be missed if you're not looking. Pituitary cystic lesion and cerebellum/brainstem lacunar infarcts may be more conspicuous on T2 than other sequences.
    - Make sure the check the marrow signal not just of the vertebral bodies but also the pedicles/posterior elements, skull base, and bony pelvis.
    - Do not forget the bony pelvis and sacroiliac joints. It extremely easy to miss pathology at these sites. (Dictation macros do not often mention this region, even though it is seen frequently on lumbar imaging – a potential modification to prevent error.)
    - It can be very easy to pass epidural collections, dismissing them as normal CSF when they are T2 hyperintense. Make sure to look carefully at cord morphology/displacement, and to always correlate any conceivable T2 hyperintense structure across all sequences. Looking carefully for cord displacement can also help you detect herniation, web, arachnoid cysts, etc.

- T1 Post contrast.
    - Most people will detect abnormal intraspinal enhancement. Make sure you look closely at the paraspinal soft tissues and neuroforamina as well, as these are blind spots.
    - The paraspinal musculature, especially the iliacus and psoas muscles are frequently involved in spinal infection and even neoplastic/infiltrative disease. Don't forget to check for involvement of these sights.

- Miscellaneous.
  - Note that differing sequences may image different anatomy, especially if the patient moves during an exam (even the position of the sat band can change). This can unveil new anatomy and pathology.
  - Imaging in the differing planes often covers different anatomy. Check the edges/corners on every sequence.
  - Be extremely careful about numbering the vertebra. It's best to not assume the usual number of cervical, thoracic, or lumbar vertebra. Segmentation anomalies such as extra ribs, transitional lumbosacral anatomy, and fused vertebra can confuse the picture. Remain consistent with prior reports, and use numbering from C1-C2 through the spine as the gold standard.
    - When the numbering of lumbar levels is unclear, we'll use wording such as "The last well-formed disc space will be considered L5-S1 for the purposes of this study."
    - It can sometimes be useful to say: "Recommend confirmation of spinal level prior to any invasive procedure by imaging the whole spine and numbering from the craniocervical junction."

Search Patterns for Acute/Vascular Exams

Long H. Tu

Mehmet Emin Adin

Sandra Abi Fadel

MRA Brain

MRA brain studies are performed to evaluate/follow aneurysms, stenosis/occlusion, and other vascular abnormalities.

It's important to remember that you can make out the brain and a lot of non-vascular anatomy even on MRA TOF sequences. This portion is mostly suppressed, so there is a temptation to not look at all. You will occasionally find mass lesions, prior infarct/hemorrhage, and other significant findings. Below is an example step by step approach.

- Check the indication, history, and priors.
    - Especially look at any prior CTA head and neck as well as recent MRI brain.
    - Know if there are previously detected aneurysms/vascular abnormalities and any prior treatment or complication.

- Examine the localizer images.
    - As usually, be especially careful to check the anatomy that may not be covered by the cross-sectional images.

- Examine the diffusion weighted images (if obtained).
    - If no conventional MR sequences are obtained besides the MRA, remember that the B0 DWI images can be used as a "poor man's" susceptibility imaging.
    - Window tightly and scroll slowly, image by image, to look for stroke, especially if there is a recent/acute neurologic presentation.
    - You'll occasionally see a new/recent infarct on routine follow up for aneurysms, so make sure to look closely every time!

- Assess the arterial vasculature on the TOF images.
    - It is useful to MPR thin/raw images into coronal and sagittal. Thin reconstructions are particularly helpful to detect subtle abnormality at certain segments, e.g., the carotid siphons and supraclinoid segments.

- It can be very useful to screen the anatomy quickly with thicker slice MIP or average-projection images. Use at least two projections for every anatomic segment of a vessel. Axials and coronals will usually suffice for the whole circle of Willis. Coronals are particularly useful to assess the posterior circulation. Compare overall vessel density on thick MIPs, which can help you detect more subtle or distal occlusions.
- At each vessel, look for narrowing, loss of signal, and abnormal/additional vessels.
- I generally prefer to look for aneurysms specifically on additional second pass, focusing on branch points where they are most common. Note that carotid terminus, basilar tip, and posterior circulation branchpoint aneurysms are easy to miss on axial projections. Be particularly careful to look at these sites carefully on the coronal images.
- You can look at the vessels in any order you'd like as long as you cover all of them. Here is the order of vessels I usually do. I start with the anterior circulation, assessing primarily with axial and coronal images:
    - Right ICA (incidental upper cervical and intracranial), MCA, and ACA.
    - Left ICA (incidental upper cervical and intracranial), MCA, and ACA.
- Then I look at the posterior circulation, using mostly coronals, correlating with axials and sagittals as needed.
    - Right vertebral (incidental upper cervical and intracranial) and PICA.
    - Left vertebral (incidental upper cervical and intracranial) and PICA.
    - Basilar artery.
    - Right SCA and PCA.
    - Left SCA and PCA.
- Note that as with other vascular imaging, the most common missed stenoses and occlusions are in the distal MCA beyond the M1 segment (usually M2). Make sure to distinguish each ACA, as it can be difficult to detect a cut off if there is significant tortuosity. Distinguish the PCA from

the ipsilateral SCAs and/or basal vein of Rosenthal (if visualized).
    - Corroborate any abnormality with prior CTA/MRA or even MRI brain.

- If you have an aneurysm, and are looking for flow related signal in residual lumen, be careful to check any available T1 sequences to make sure that you do not confuse inherent T1 (i.e., blood product) for flow related signal and misinterpret as persistent lumen.

- If you have post-contrast images, repeat the same search pattern, though with special attention to any areas of previously identified abnormality, or prior aneurysm coiling/clipping.

- Remember to at least quickly look at the non-vascular anatomy.
    - This is especially important if the patient does not have a recent comparison CT/MRI.
    - Use a similar search pattern as you would for other brain/head imaging, e.g., scalp/soft tissues, bones, CSF spaces, and brain.

- Last checks.
    - MRA brain is often used to follow the course of known aneurysms. Be wary of the temptation to merely compare the known abnormalities and move on. Patients with aneurysms are likely to have more than one and are predisposed to form new aneurysms. Look especially careful to additional new or previously missed abnormalities. You may find occasional instances of prior "satisfaction of search" errors.
    - Even if the patient had a recent similar MRA or equivalent study CTA or DSA, remember to look as if you are the first reader because the prior read may have missed aneurysms due to satisfaction of search by a more acute or more impressive abnormality.

- Remember to proofread.

Vessel Wall Imaging

Vessel wall imaging (VWI) is an increasingly used modality to assess stroke mechanism, and to characterize/identify vasculitis, dissections, Moyamoya, and aneurysms. Usually the abnormality is already known (or you're looking for a diffuse process), so it is not a challenge to find the abnormality. Below is a quick primer on expected imaging appearance in varying conditions and practical checklist for clinical practice.

Imaging Findings

Indication	Enhancement	NO Enhancement	Notes
Aneurysm	Higher risk for rupture (or recently ruptured)	Likely incidental or lower risk, though not very specific	VWI can be used to localize the culprit/bleeding aneurysm in patients with multiple aneurysms
Atherosclerotic plaque	Focal/eccentric enhancement = vulnerable plaque	Lower risk	If you see *circumferential* enhancement (especially without stenosis), consider other vasculopathies
Vasculitis	Higher yield for biopsy (active inflammation)	Low yield of biopsy	Usually circumferential enhancement. If focal/eccentric, consider instead atherosclerosis
Vessel narrowing DDX: RCVS vs vasculitis	More likely vasculitis	More likely RCVS (also allowed minimal enhancement)	RCVS is also expected to resolve over time
Moyamoya	If concentric, more likely secondary causes of moyamoya	More likely primary Moyamoya (allowed thin/mild enhancemnet)	If enhancement is focal/eccentric and outward remodeling, consider atherosclerosis

Checklist/Search Pattern for VWI

Review the indication, history, and prior studies.

- Where is the suspected abnormality?
- What are the suspected etiologies for which the study is being performed?
- Does the patient have a systemic vasculitis, inflammatory condition, or other predisposing factor for intracranial vasculopathy?
- Has the patient received corticosteroids, which can decrease/eliminate vessel wall enhancement?
- Where is the site of any recent occlusion/recanalization or thrombectomy?
- Has there been recent MR contrast administration (<12h), which can produce spurious signal?
- Look at all vessels of concern on prior MRA/angiographic imaging. Don't forget prior catheter angiograms/DSA.

Assess technique:

- Knowing the site of suspected abnormality will help you chose the area of interest (FOV) if using 2D technique.
- If looking for a diffuse process, choose planes that include as much of circle of Willis as possible. If expecting a peripheral/small artery process, include small branches of the intracranial vessels as well. 3D acquisition may helpful if this is available.

Checklist for interpretation.

- Remember that this can be used for both intracranial and extracranial vessels.
- Look for vessel wall enhancement.
    - Look at all vessels on the images for multifocal processes, e.g., right then left ICAs, and proximal MCAs, ACAs, and PCAs.
    - Look for abnormal enhancement extending to perivascular tissues (can be seen vasculitis).
- Pitfalls:
    - Normal wall enhancement can be seen where ICAs and vertebral arteries cross the dura.
    - Slow flow in vessels or veins near arteries can mimic vessel wall enhancement. Check on multiple planes.

- In atherosclerosis, look for juxta-luminal fibrous cab (bright signal in otherwise blacked-out lumen).
- Prominent vasa vasorum can be seen in older patients with extensive atherosclerosis, mimicking pathologic enhancement.

References:

1. Young CC, Bonow RH, Barros G, Mossa-Basha M, Kim LJ, Levitt MR. Magnetic resonance vessel wall imaging in cerebrovascular diseases. Neurosurgical focus. 2019 Dec 1;47(6):E4.
2. Lindenholz A, van der Kolk AG, Zwanenburg JJ, Hendrikse J. The use and pitfalls of intracranial vessel wall imaging: how we do it. Radiology. 2018 Jan;286(1):12-28.
3. Mandell DM, Mossa-Basha M, Qiao Y, Hess CP, Hui F, Matouk C, Johnson MH, Daemen MJ, Vossough A, Edjlali M, Saloner D. Intracranial vessel wall MRI: principles and expert consensus recommendations of the American Society of Neuroradiology. American Journal of Neuroradiology. 2017 Feb 1;38(2):218-29.
4. Santarosa C, Cord B, Koo A, Bhogal P, Malhotra A, Payabvash S, Minja FJ, Matouk CC. Vessel wall magnetic resonance imaging in intracranial aneurysms: principles and emerging clinical applications. Interventional Neuroradiology. 2020 Apr;26(2):135-46.

MRA Neck

The MRA neck with and without contrast is often used to assess for dissection. It also has utility in the assessment of high-grade stenosis, vascular malformations, anatomic variation, and subclavian steal. The approach is straightforward, first assessing the vessels with the TOF angiographic images, then the post-contrast MRA sequence. A portion of the upper thoracic as well as intracranial vasculature may be incidentally seen, so it is important to look at these as well. Then, you can use the fat saturated T1 images to look for dissection/intramural hematoma. These sequences can also be used to look for peri-vascular inflammation or adjacent soft tissue abnormality. Like with MRA of the brain, many non-vascular structures will be incidentally imaged. It's important to at least take a quick look at these. Below is a suggested approach:

- Check the indication, history, and priors.
    - Especially look at any prior CTA head and neck as well as recent MRI brain. Know the location of any recent infarcts, recent traumatic injuries, or other potentially relevant pathologies.

- Examine the localizer images
    - As usually, be especially careful to check the anatomy that may not be covered by the cross-sectional images.

- Assess the arterial vasculature on the TOF images.
    - Rather than examining everything on only the axials, it can be more efficient to use an MPR viewer. Reorient the planes so that the vessels are laid out/in plane on the coronals then use MIPs and thick slab average projections to quickly assess each vessel. It can be helpful to take a quick look in at least two planes (e.g., coronal and sagittal), which can improve detection of lesions.
    - At each of the following, make sure to assess for narrowing, loss of signal, aneurysms, and abnormal/additional vessels, mural irregularities, or perivascular thickening (e.g., in carotidynia):
        - Aortic arch and visualized descending aorta.

        - Brachiocephalic trunk.
        - Right then left subclavian arteries (follow these to the edge of the study).
        - Right then left common carotid arteries, proximal external carotid arteries (and branches), then internal carotid arteries.
        - Right then left vertebral arteries.
    - Remember that TOF will often overestimate stenosis relative to contrast enhanced study or DSA.

- Assess any incidentally imaged intracranial arterial anatomy.
    - Look for vessel cut-offs. Check the branch points for aneurysms.
        - Right then left ICAs.
        - Right then left MCAS.
        - Right then left ACAS.
        - Right then left vertebral arteries.
        - Basilar artery.
        - Right then left SCAs.
        - Right then left PCAs.

- Examine the pre-contrast T1 sequences.
    - Look for peripheral or crescentic hyperintensity associated with the visualized upper chest, neck, and visualized intracranial arteries following a similar order/approach as for the TOF and post-contrast MRA images.
    - Look at the non-vascular structures, at least briefly, for incidental masses/lesions. Fat-specific (e.g., Dixon) sequences, if obtained, can be advantageous to detect mass lesions distorting or invading fat planes.

- Repeat the above process with any post-contrast MRA images.
    - Subtraction images may be particularly helpful at this stage. Pay special attention to areas of stenosis or abnormality seen on the TOF images, which may overestimate stenosis.
    - Note any areas that do not fill on the TOF images, but that do fill on post-contrast. These may represent slow or retrograde flow (e.g., in steal syndromes).

- Look for abnormal signal outside of the arteries on the post-contrast subtraction images, in cases where you're concerned for active hemorrhage, pseudoaneurysm, or arteriovenous fistula.
- Look at the non-vascular structures on the raw (not-subtracted) post-contrast images. Be careful to at least quickly run your search pattern for the neck through these images. This includes examining the intracranial compartment, neck soft tissues, mucosal surfaces, facial structures, supraclavicular fossae, upper mediastinum, lungs, chest wall, and osseous structures.

- Proofread.

MRV Brain

MRV brain is the gold standard to detect venous sinus thrombosis. Thrombus demonstrates complex and unpredictable changes in T1 and T2/FLAIR signal as it evolves from acute to chronic stage. Clot may also enhance in the subacute/chronic phase. Therefore, conventional MRI is not highly sensitive/specific for chronic venous thrombosis. Convention MRI with pre- and post-contrast 3D T1 is generally sufficient to exclude acute/subacute thrombus.

The best conventional sequence is usually post-contrast MPRAGE (3D GRE) compared to pre-contrast T1/MPRAGE. This will detect most acute/subacute thrombus. However, thrombus that enhances or is at a phase with higher inherent T1 signal may be occult to post-contrast MPRAGE. The most sensitive imaging sequences for acute thrombus therefore are dynamic post-contrast MR venogram, where you can see a filling defect as contrast first fills the sinus. At our institution, we do MR venogram with and without contrast, along with MPRAGE and diffusion weighted images to look for infarct.

The MR venogram images (especially late dynamic post-contrast) images can show incidental non-vascular pathology. This is also true of any currently obtained MPRAGE images, even if a concurrent full MR brain is not obtained. Make sure to at least look quickly at these sets of images for incidental, and potentially significant pathology.

- Check the indication, history, and priors.
    - Especially look at any prior CTA head and neck as well as recent MRI brain. The venous sinuses often opacify on CTA exams, which can prime you to any expected abnormality.

- Assess adequacy/technique.
    - If the patient cannot receive contrast, obtaining a concurrent conventional MRI brain, for T1, T2/FLAIR, and SWI sequences can help increase sensitivity compared to just a TOF sequence.
    - 3D phase contrast (PC) MRV is another technique that can used if a patient cannot receive contrast, and is superior to 2D TOF MRV.

- If the above cannot be done, 2D TOF MRV in multiple planes/projections can help clarify areas of artifact that occur when the direction of flow is in the plane of imaging. Actively monitoring the study can be useful to choose the direction expected to resolve potential artifact.

- Examine the localizer images.
    - As usually, be especially careful to check the anatomy that may not be covered by the cross-sectional images.
    - Take a quick look at the brain parenchyma, especially if there is not a concordant brain MRI.

- Examine the diffusion weighted images as usual.
    - You'll want to look for secondary brain edema, infarct, and hemorrhage if there is a venous thrombosis.
    - Note that if you do not have conventional T2/FLAIR sequences, that DWI can used to see larger regions of brain edema (as T2 shine through).
    - Note that not all, even true restricted diffusion with venous thrombosis is infarct. Some may reflect severe brain edema, and may be reversible with anticoagulation/treatment.
    - Remember that the B0 images can detect susceptibility artifact, in the case that you do not have conventional SWI.

- First assess TOF images, which can give you a sense of the overall anatomy.
    - It can be difficult to differentiate thrombosis from a hypoplastic sinus on TOF images, though comparison to priors may be helpful if there are only non-contrast/TOF MRV images.
    - If there are no post-contrast MRV images, apply the below search pattern to the TOF/PC sequence.

- Using post contrast MRV images, look for thrombus/filling at the:
    - Deep system.
        - Superior sagittal sinus.
        - Inferior sagittal sinus.
        - Internal (and other deep) cerebral veins.

        - Vein of Galen.
        - Straight sinus.
        - Confluence of the sinuses.
        - Right then left transverse and sigmoid sinuses.
        - Exiting jugular veins.
        - Cavernous sinus.
        - Superior and inferior petrosal sinuses.
    - Other/superficial veins (as able, usually less well seen, unless thrombosed):
        - Ophthalmic veins.
        - Cortical veins.
        - Vein of Labbe.
        - Vein of Trolard.
    - Be careful of anatomic variations at the confluence of the sinuses. Do not "over call" thrombosis when there is an early bifurcation in the transverse sinuses or areas of developmental hypoplasia.
    - Variants are important especially when MRV is done pre-operatively. Prescence/position of an occipital sinus should be mentioned if the patient is planned for posterior fossa surgery.
    - Consider the sizes of the transverse, sigmoid and jugular bulb. Hypoplasia of these usually occurs together on the left or right. If only one of these is small on a side, be more suspicious for thrombus.
    - You can also apply the above search pattern to any post-contrast MPRAGE sequence. Note that you'll need a pre-contrast T1/MPRAGE to exclude thrombus with inherent T1 similar to post-contrast signal.

- On dynamic post-contrast images, you may incidentally see the whole of the arterial vasculature.
    - Going time point by time point, make sure to look at the arterial system, if captured. Assess the upper cervical ICAs/vertebral arteries, MCAs, ACAs, vertebrobasilar system and PCAs.
    - Look for vessel cut-off and high-grade stenosis.
    - Look for aneurysm.

- Look for vascular malformation/early venous filling.
- You are liable for arterial findings if you're provided these images!

- Look for nonvascular findings:
  - Look for any narrowing of the venous sinuses (especially the lateral transverse sinuses). You may see associated findings of idiopathic intracranial hypertension incidentally on the MPRAGE or other sequences. You might also suggest the diagnosis and recommend clinical correlation or further imaging.
  - No matter what imaging sequences you have, do a quick search of the nonvascular anatomy. For non-contrast MRV, this may be the TOF images. For contrast enhanced MRV, the non-vascular anatomy is often best seen on later post-contrast dynamic MRV and/or post-contrast MPRAGE (if obtained).

- Remember to correlate any abnormalities with prior studies.

- Remember to proofread.

References:

1. Canedo-Antelo M, Baleato-González S, Mosqueira AJ, Casas-Martínez J, Oleaga L, Vilanova JC, Luna-Alcalá A, García-Figueiras R. Radiologic clues to cerebral venous thrombosis. RadioGraphics. 2019 Oct;39(6):1611-28.
2. Leach JL, Fortuna RB, Jones BV, Gaskill-Shipley MF. Imaging of cerebral venous thrombosis: current techniques, spectrum of findings, and diagnostic pitfalls. Radiographics. 2006 Oct;26(suppl_1):S19-41.

CT Perfusion for Stroke

CT perfusion (CTP) is often done concurrent with CTA head and neck imaging to select patients for reperfusion. There are some helpful articles and videos to give you a foundation in what this technique entails, which I've referenced at the end. I would recommend at least getting a knowledge base in this topic early in fellowship if you don't have it already. There are several software packages for automatic perfusion abnormality processing and quantification. At our institution, we use RAPID, so this section is written with reference to that workflow. Below is a checklist/process I use for every study.

- Check the indication, history, and priors.
    - Know what the presentation is, and consider where the predicted lesion or hypoperfusion may be.
    - Note if the patient had a recent (iodine) contrast enhanced study. This can compromise the accuracy of the exam.
    - The CT perfusion can often clue you in to abnormalities that you'll expect on the CTA head and neck. If these are available at the same time, I often look at the CTP first. This can help detect subtle/distal lesions.
    - It can be also useful to know if the patient has underlying cardiovascular abnormalities or alterations in the intracranial anatomy/pressure that could alter contrast bolus delivery kinetics. Interpretation of the study has to take place within this context.

- Assess study adequacy.
    - Check the AIF and VOF functions.
        - These should both have swift/sharp upstroke and sharp (single) peaks.
        - AIF peak ideally >200 HU. AIF peak >80-100 HU may still be diagnostic, depending on the other study factors.
        - VOF should be higher and have larger area under the curve than AIF.
        - Both curves should return to near baseline in less than 50 seconds.
    - Check the ROI placement for the AIF and VOF functions.
        - AIF should be on a proximal artery (e.g., M1 MCA). Ideally away from any known abnormality. The

basilar artery is any option the case of bilateral anterior disease.
    - VOF should be on a large venous structure (e.g., SSS or confluence of sinuses).
  - Assess for motion.
    - Scroll through the "shuttle" series, i.e., raw data, to see if the patient moved during the study. This can compromise the dynamic information you see in the curves and perfusion maps.
    - Reprocessing may be able remove limitations of motion in the first 10-15 seconds, as long as you still have a few seconds of baseline before the AIF and VOF peaks.
  - Troubleshoot any issues with the above.
    - You can either manually process the study using an institutional link or call an IT help line.
    - A common issue is that AIF and VOF ROIs are erroneous in placement. Other times, the study is sufficiently limited that the perfusion maps cannot be corrected, and you'll have to interpret the study within these limitations.
- Examine the perfusion maps.
  - Quantify and report the following values:
    - The infarct core (approximated by CBV<30mL).
    - The core + penumbra: delayed MTT (>6s)
    - The mismatch volume, (i.e., ischemic penumbra, tissue at risk): the difference in the areas of hypoperfusion (>6s) and infarct core above.
    - The mismatch ratio = (core + penumbra) / core.
  - Look at the MTT maps for other areas of hypoperfusion which may not meet the above threshold.
    - Areas of delayed transit not meeting the >6s threshold, may be artifactual, but can sometimes indicate areas that will soon be ischemic.
    - Especially if these match an expected area of ischemia from the clinical presentation or concurrent CTA findings, consider reporting this within context as suspicious for that may subsequently be at risk. Consider follow up imaging by MRI/CTP.

    - Note that the commonly used CBV and MTT cut offs are chosen as at a balance of sensitivity and specificity. These may not always have exact correlation with infarct core/penumbra.

- Remember to report any findings within context of presentation, cardiovascular status/study limitations, and if possible, findings of concurrent CT/CTA.

- Proofread.

References:

1. Wing, Stevan Christopher, and Hugh S. Markus. "Interpreting CT perfusion in stroke." Practical neurology 19.2 (2019): 136-142.
2. Demeestere, Jelle, et al. "Review of perfusion imaging in acute ischemic stroke: from time to tissue." Stroke 51.3 (2020): 1017-1024.

MR Perfusion for Stroke

MR perfusion (MRP) for stroke or ischemia is less commonly performed than CT, in part related to availability and speed of access. There are some circumstances where this sort of study will be performed instead such as contraindication to CT contrast. The approach is similar to as with CTP, with some minor variations. The most important difference is the infarct core is delineated by ADC value rather than CBV. For patients who cannot receive contrast, arterial spin labeled MR perfusion may be an option, based on institutional availability.

- Check the indication, history, and priors.
    - Know what the presentation is, and consider where the predicted lesion or hypoperfusion may be.
    - Note if the patient had a recent (gadolinium) contrast enhanced study. This can compromise the accuracy of the exam.
    - It can be also useful to know if the patient has underlying cardiovascular abnormalities or alterations in the intracranial anatomy/pressure that could alter contrast bolus delivery kineties. Interpretation of the study has to take place within this context.

- Assess study adequacy.
    - Check the AIF and VOF functions.
        - These should both have swift/sharp upstroke and sharp (single) peaks.
        - AIF peak >100 a.u. may be adequate for most studies.
        - VOF should be higher and have larger area under the curve than AIF.
        - Both curves should return to near baseline in less than 50 seconds.
    - Check the ROI placement for the AIF and VOF functions.
        - AIF should be on a proximal artery (e.g., M1 MCA)
        - VOF should be on a large venous structure (e.g., SSS or confluence of sinuses).
    - Assess for motion.
        - Scroll through the "shuttle" series, i.e. raw data, to see if the patient moved during the study. This can compromise the dynamic information you see in the

curves and perfusion maps. Reprocessing may resolve minor issues.

- Troubleshoot any issues with the above.
  - You can either manually process the study using an institutional link or call an IT help line.
  - A common issue is that AIF and VOF ROIs are erroneous in placement. Other times, the study is sufficiently limited that the perfusion maps cannot be corrected, and you'll have to interpret the study within these limitations.

- Examine the perfusion maps.
  - Quantify and report the following values:
    - The infarct core (approximated by ADC<620mL).
    - The core + penumbra: delayed MTT (>6s)
    - The mismatch volume, (i.e., ischemic penumbra, tissue at risk): the difference in the areas of hypoperfusion (>6s) and infarct core above.
    - The mismatch ratio = (core + penumbra) / core.
  - Look at the MTT maps for other areas of hypoperfusion which may not meet the about threshold.
    - Areas of delayed transit not meeting the >6s threshold, may be artifactual, but can sometimes indicate areas that will soon be ischemic.
    - Especially if these match an expected area of ischemia from the clinical presentation or concurrent MRA/MRI findings, consider reporting this within context as suspicious for that may subsequently be at risk. Consider follow up imaging by MRI/MRP.
  - Note that the commonly used ADC and MTT cut offs are chosen as at a balance of sensitivity and specificity. These may not always have exact correlation with infarct core/penumbra.

- Remember to report any findings within context of presentation, cardiovascular status/study limitations, and if possible, findings of concurrent MRI/MRV.

- Proofread.

References:

1. Heit JJ, Wintermark M. Perfusion computed tomography for the evaluation of acute ischemic stroke: strengths and pitfalls. Stroke. 2016 Apr;47(4):1153-8.

Search Patterns for Uncommon MRI Exams

Long H. Tu

Sam Payabvash

Ichiro Ikuta

MRI Brachial Plexus

The brachial plexus MRI can be intimidating because of the underlying complexity of the brachial plexus nerve connections. In interpreting a brachial plexus MRI however, much of that complexity does not always have to be immediately recalled. It is useful to have a general sense of where each segment is located, i.e., roots, trunks, divisions, cords, and branches (mnemonic: "rad techs drink cold beverages"). If there is an abnormality, then you should look up the exact underlying anatomy as needed. The overall approach is made simpler this way.

You can start reading the study like an MRI cervical spine. Once you are done looking at the spinal anatomy and spinal canal, you'll follow the nerve roots into the soft tissues of the neck, where they become the brachial plexus. You'll trace the plexus between the anterior and middle scalene muscles, the follow the remaining course near the subclavian vessels, to the edge of the study in the upper arm. You'll be looking for the sorts of pathology that would affect nerves anywhere in the body: mass lesions, infection/inflammation, abnormal thickening/enhancement, etc. Lastly, you'll assess the muscles of the imaged upper chest/arm for secondary denervation, and then all the other osseous, vascular, etc. anatomy for incidentals.

Of note, the brachial plexus is easily identified peripherally due to its close association with the subclavian vessels. Some neuroradiologists will start peripherally and then trace the plexus medially for this reason.

Like with other MRI exams, it can help with orientation to hang all the coronals together, all the axials together, and all the sagittal together. Coronals tend to lay the brachial plexus out well (some institutions will provide oblique coronals for optimal imaging). Sagittals provide a cross section, especially more centrally. Axials are useful for problem solving and for a cross-section at the inferior most imaged aspects. A suggested checklist approach is below:

- Check the indication, history, and priors.
    - Note the brachial plexus will be seen on prior imaging of the neck or chest, including CT and PET/CT. Neck and chest x-rays are useful to look for cervical ribs. There will also be overlapping anatomy on any prior CT/MRI of the shoulder or upper arm.

    - Check the electronic medical record for any electromyogram/nerve conduction studies (EMG/NCS), which can help localize expected abnormalities.

- Examine the localizers.
    - Be especially careful to look at anatomy that might not be covered by the cross-sectional images.

- Examine the visualized cervical spine in usual fashion.
    - Assess the alignment, vertebral body heights, discs, intraspinal compartment, neuroforamina, etc.
    - Specifically examine the course of each of the exiting nerve roots in the neuroforamina on the side of the imaged brachial plexus (if not both sides).
    - Look for pseudomeningoceles and other collections/masses at the neuroforamen.
    - Note that incidental spine pathology/degeneration may ultimately account for the patient's symptoms even when a plexopathy is suspected.

- Examine the brachial plexus nerves.
    - On each sequence, follow the nerves (roots) from the neuroforamina through the anterior and middle scalene muscles (trunks). The nerves then course in the suprascapular region then posterior to the clavicle (divisions). Follow the plexus inferior to the clavicle (cords), and then past the lateral border of the pectoralis minor muscle/coracoid process (branches).
        - The coronal view usually lays out the whole plexus well.
        - The sagittal view of often best to assess more central portions of the plexus in cross section. Axial images can be used more peripherally.
    - On T1: Look for loss of fat plane with the brachial plexus, haziness of fat, mass effect, and anatomic distortion. This may relate to a lung apical mass, lymph node, or mass lesion in neck. Quickly assess the normal fat planes of the lateral

neck. Using all three planes, look for abnormal effacement of the fat, abnormal nerve root thickening.
    - On T2 FS/STIR, look for edema and inflammation involving the brachial plexus and branches. MR neurography may optimize nerve evaluation.
    - On T1 post contrast, look for abnormal enhancement, mass lesions, etc. around the brachial plexus.
    - For regional or diffuse processes, it can be useful to refer to the plexus in supraclavicular, clavicular, or infraclavicular segments (or alternatively medial, mid, or distal). If a single component of the brachial plexus is involved, then more detailed anatomic discussion could ensue.

- Examine the visualized musculature.
    - On T1, look for loss of bulk and/or fatty atrophy.
    - On T2 FS/STIR, look for muscle edema (post-traumatic or denervation).
    - On T1 post contrast, look for abnormal muscle enhancement.
    - Depending the pattern of muscle involvement, you should suspect a lesion at a particular part of the brachial plexus or surrounding shoulder. For example:
        - Deltoid and teres minor – axillary nerve (consider also quadrilateral space syndrome).
        - Supraspinatus/infraspinatus - suprascapular nerve (look for suprascapular notch or spinoglenoid notch lesion or consider Parsonage Turner syndrome)
        - Brachialis, biceps brachii and coracobrachialis – musculocutaneous nerve (C5, C6, and C7).
        - Triceps – radial nerve (possible triangular interval lesion).
        - Muscles in the forearm and hand, innervated by other branches of the brachial plexus are often not seen within the study field of view. Any denervation changes would have to be inferred from clinical notes or other imaging.

- Assess the remaining osseous anatomy.
    - On T1, look for preserved marrow signal. Look for cortical discontinuity. Look for formational/segmentation abnormalities:
        - E.g., cervical ribs, large transverse processes at C7, abnormal shape/pseudoarthrosis of the first rib with the second.
    - On T2 FS/STIR, look for marrow edema.
    - On T1 post contrast, look for abnormal marrow, periosteal, and periarticular enhancement.

- Assess the glenohumeral and acromioclavicular joints to the extent able.
    - Joint pathology may simulate/contribute to symptoms prompting imaging of the brachial plexus.
    - Look for any joint effusion, obvious/large rotator cuff tear, severe degeneration or deformity. These are usefully best seen with fluid-sensitive sequences (T2 with fat sat or STIR).
    - If needed, recommend MRI shoulder.

- Examine the visceral and soft tissues.
    - Make sure to look at the visualized lung and mediastinum, especially for adenopathy and mass lesions. Remember to look at the lung apex/superior sulcus.
    - Make sure to look at the major arteries and veins, especially for occlusion, stenosis, and mass effect.
    - Look for any axillary lymphadenopathy.
    - Look for any subcutaneous and cutaneous lesions.

- Proofread.

References:

1. Gilcrease-Garcia BM, Deshmukh SD, Parsons MS. Anatomy, imaging, and pathologic conditions of the brachial plexus. RadioGraphics. 2020 Oct;40(6):1686-714.
2. Castillo M. Imaging the anatomy of the brachial plexus: review and self-assessment module. American Journal of Roentgenology. 2005 Dec;185(6_supplement):S196-204.
3. Michigan State University Department of Radiology Lecture: The Brachial Plexus. https://youtu.be/zJFpHQQoiG8. Accessed May 16, 2021.

MRI Thoracic Outlet Syndrome

Thoracic outlet syndrome (TOS) can be neurogenic, arterial, or venous in etiology. Neurogenic TOS is usually a clinical diagnosis, with imaging corroboration most appropriate via brachial plexus MRI (extrinsic compression/edema of nerves). Vascular TOS may be evaluated by MRI, usually with a combination of dynamic post-contrast sequences and traditional post-contrast images, often 3D GRE/T1. The same sequences are done with arms lowered and arms raised. At our institution, this protocol is added to the brachial plexus study or performed as a separate exam when there is concern for vascular thoracic outlet syndrome. Below is a suggested approach:

- Check the indication, history, and priors.
    - Know what the patient's symptoms are and what side they are on. This can give you a sense as to whether there is likely arterial or venous pathology and where you should look especially closely.
    - Use prior imaging to assess the presence of lines/intravascular devices. Know if there are surgical clips or hardware that will produce susceptibility on MRI. Cervical ribs or nearby fractures can be seen on chest x-ray, cervical spine CT, PET/CT, etc.

- Assess technique/adequacy.
    - The IV injection site should be on the asymptomatic or less symptomatic side.
    - Look for any artifact that will limit the evaluation of vessels.

- Assess the dynamic post-contrast images.
    - We generally look at the arms lowered images first then look at the arms raised images after.

- Follow the contrast bolus from the central/arterial phase, image-by-image, through the parenchymal/venous phase, and through the return of contrast centrally. The general order of vessels is:
    - Aorta.
    - Brachiocephalic trunk.
    - Common carotid arteries.
    - Subclavian and axillary arteries.
    - Vertebral arteries (as able).
    - Internal and external jugular veins.
    - Axillary, subclavian, and brachiocephalic veins.
    - Superior vena cava.
- On each image, look for:
    - Thrombosis (both arterial and venous).
        - Arterial thrombus may sometimes be well demonstrated on venous phase images, when the expanded wall enhances around the thrombus.
    - Vessel narrowing or irregularity.
    - Enlarged collaterals (may be along neck/chest wall).
    - Vessel wall thickening.
    - Aneurysms/pseudoaneurysms (both arterial and venous).
    - Perivascular inflammation.
    - Note that incidental imaging of pulmonary artery (or other vascular) pathology can clue you into systemic vasculopathies, such as Takayasu's arteritis.
- Note that reconstruction of acquired images (coronal at our institution for faster image acquisition) into axial and sagittal projections can be useful to troubleshoot questionable findings.
- Look for worsening of any pathology on the arms raised images. Obviously, look especially carefully where the vessels enter the upper chest, around the first rib, and scalene triangle (between anterior and middle scalene muscles) – common sites of compression.

- Correlate any findings with bone and soft tissue abnormalities. These are best seen on conventional brachial plexus MRI (non-contrast T1 weighted images) or prior CT/radiographic imaging. Look especially for:
    - Cervical ribs.
    - Prominent transverse process at C7.
    - Anomalous 1st rib / clavicle.
    - Soft tissue and bone mass lesions.

- Consider correlation with CT or other modalities as needed if delineation of osseous/soft tissues is not clear.

- Note that arterial/venous narrowing by itself is not diagnostic of TOS. The patient must have concordant symptoms, as many of the above findings may be seen with asymptomatic patients.

- Review for incidental findings. Given the extent of coverage, you may need to check for lymphadenopathy in the mediastinum, inferior neck, and axilla; pulmonary or paraspinal masses; thyroid gland nodules; bone tumors; etc.

- Proofread.

References:

1. Raptis CA, Sridhar S, Thompson RW, Fowler KJ, Bhalla S. Imaging of the patient with thoracic outlet syndrome. *RadioGraphics.* 2016 Jul;36(4):984-1000.

MRI Lumbosacral Plexus

MRI of the lumbosacral plexus can be an intimidating exam. The nerve anatomy is often not covered in medical school (or residency!) and it is an uncommon exam, not seen frequently even at the fellowship level. The purpose of this section is *not* to provide an exhaustive discussion the topic, but rather to demystify and organize the approach. It's recommended that you read the selected/curated references to familiarize yourself with anatomy and potential pathology if this is a wholly unfamiliar topic.

In short, the lumbosacral plexus is basically a confluence of nerves from T12 through S4. It is located in the paraspinal area in the inferior abdomen and pelvis and gives rise to three major branches. These should be familiar: 1) the sciatic nerve, which courses posterolaterally, then down the posterior leg 2) the femoral nerve, which courses between the psoas and iliacus muscles then follows the femoral vessels down the anterior leg, and 3) the obturator nerve, which courses first along the periphery of the pelvis, then medially to supply the obturators and leg adductors. The obturator nerve is the smallest of these and might not always be seen well.

Evaluation of the lumbosacral plexus comes down to first evaluating the lumbar spine and exiting nerve roots, similar as to the more common lumbar spine MRI. Next, you'll follow the nerve roots laterally to the "plexus." Then, you look where the three major branches course for pathology. If relevant, you can look along the *expected* course of smaller branches of the lumbar plexus for lesions/abnormality, even if the nerve is too small to see clearly. You'll also look for secondary findings in the musculature (such as denervation edema or fatty atrophy) and incidental pathology in the pelvis and other surrounding structures (traumatic fractures, metastatic lymphadenopathy, etc.). That covers the major steps.

Below is a step-by-step approach that can simplify this seemly complex study:

- Check the indication/history/priors.
    - Look for prior studies that may have included the lumbar/sacral spine, including prior CT/MRI of the abdomen and pelvis.
    - PET/CTs may be particularly helpful in oncologic patients.

- Don't forget to look at the localizers.
    - Be especially careful to look carefully at anatomy that is not imaged in the confines of the cross-sectional images.

- Examine the visualized lumbar spine first using a usual approach.
    - If the lumbar and sacral spine have not previously been imaged, consider discussing usual features of vertebral alignment, vertebral body height, and any marrow abnormalities.
    - It will be essential to discuss disc disease that impinges on the cord or descending/exiting nerve roots.
    - Symptoms thought to arise from pathology of the plexus may be related to more common spondylosis and spinal stenosis.

- Examine the lumbosacral plexus.
    - Consider a broad overview using STIR or T2 fat sat images to look for major asymmetry, diffuse processes, and extent of any disease.
        - Look for gross pathology along the course of the plexus from the psoas muscles, at the pelvic sidewalls, and into the bilateral inguinal regions.
        - Survey the gluteal musculature adjacent to the pelvis on axial and coronal sequences.
    - Assess the T1 pre-contrast sequences.
        - Look for mass lesions or other distortion along the plexus. Check first along the nerve roots, then along the three major branches: sciatic, obturator, and femoral.
            - Following the femoral nerve may be easiest starting peripherally, at the inguinal region next to the femoral artery/vein (rather than starting from L2-L4).
            - For the sciatic nerve, try to find it traversing the greater sciatic foramen.
        - In the appropriate setting (e.g., referable symptoms), look along the expected courses of smaller nerve branches, in particular the genitofemoral and lateral femoral cutaneous nerves.
            - The genitofemoral nerve originates from the L1-2 segments of the plexus, pierces the

psoas major and emerges from its anterior surface and gives rise to genital and femoral branches.

- The lateral femoral cutaneous nerve emerges from the lateral border of the psoas major crosses the iliacus muscle obliquely, passing under the inguinal ligament.

▪ Along each of these branches, look for abnormal masses, compression, and scarring. Look for abnormal nerve size/expansion.

o Assess the STIR/T2 fat sat (or other fluid sensitive) sequence.

▪ Assess the nerves for abnormal signal (e.g., edema) or size (thickening). Look at the adjacent fat planes for abnormal fluid signal/inflammation.

▪ As previously, look along the nerve roots, then along the three major branches: sciatic, obturator, and femoral nerves.

- Look for asymmetry between the piriformis muscles and sciatic nerves if there is concern for "piriformis syndrome." Follow the course of the sciatic nerve relative to the piriformis muscle (which can be variable).

▪ In the appropriate setting (e.g., referable symptoms), look along the expected courses of smaller nerve branches, e.g., the genitofemoral and lateral femoral cutaneous nerves.

o T1 post-contrast.

▪ Look for abnormal enhancement along the visualized nerve roots, plexus, and major branches using a similar search as above.

- Assess the musculature.
    - o Look for evidence of atrophy (T1 hyperintense fat and loss of muscle bulk) or denervation edema (fluid sensitive and post-contrast sequences). Patterns of denervation implicate differing parts of the plexus.
        - ▪ Femoral nerve – hip flexors (pectineus, iliacus, sartorius) and the extensors of the knee (quadriceps femoris).

        - Sciatic nerve - posterior thigh (biceps femoris, semimembranosus and semitendinosus) and the hamstring portion of the adductor magnus.
        - Obturator nerve - muscles of the medial compartment of the thigh (obturator externus, adductor longus, adductor brevis, adductor magnus and gracilis).
    - Look for muscular avulsion injuries.
        - Avulsions most associated with nerve injury: ischial tuberosity, inferior pubic symphysis, greater trochanter.
        - Look for other pelvic avulsion that may correlate with the patient's symptoms/presentation: iliac crest, ASIS, AIIS, lesser trochanter.
    - Look for tendinopathy.
        - Look for inflammation of myotendinous junctions, partial or full-thickness tears, etc.

- Examine the remaining visceral, osseous, and soft tissue anatomy.
    - Look at each solid organ, bowel, vasculature, lymph node stations, the reproductive organs/GU tract, ureters, and bladder.
    - Make sure to assess the remaining osseous structures, including the visualized sacrum, sacroiliac joints, and femoroacetabular articulations (hips).
        - T1 pre-contrast: Look for mass lesions and loss of normal pelvic fat planes. Look for preserved signal of all visualized bones.
        - T2 FS/fluid sensitive sequences: Look for abnormal fluid collections/edema, and adenopathy.
        - T1 post-contrast: abnormal enhancement/mass lesions.
        - Sacroiliac and hip pathology can mimic lumbosacral plexopathies.
    - Look at the subcutaneous fat for incidental lesions.

- Don't forget to proofread!

References:

1. Soldatos T, Andreisek G, Thawait GK, Guggenberger R, Williams EH, Carrino JA, Chhabra A. High-resolution 3-T MR neurography of the lumbosacral plexus. Radiographics. 2013 Jul;33(4):967-87.
2. Neufeld EA, Shen PY, Nidecker AE, Runner G, Bateni C, Tse G, Chin C. MR imaging of the lumbosacral plexus: a review of techniques and pathologies. Journal of Neuroimaging. 2015 Sep;25(5):691-703.
3. Allen H, et al. MRI of the Lumbosacral Plexus: What the Practicing Radiologist Needs to Know. https://skeletalrad.org/sites/default/files/pdf/23%20-%20MRI%20of%20the%20Lumbosacral%20Plexus-%20What%20the%20Practicing%20Radiologist%20Needs%20to%20Know.pdf Accessed: 4/26/2021

MRI Temporomandibular Joints

MRI of the temporomandibular joints (MRI TMJ) is an uncommonly performed exam. It's useful to have an organized approach, as it's unlikely that you'll see enough examples in fellowship to develop an intuition for this study. The most common indications are to look for abnormalities of the disc and degenerative changes, less commonly you'll see inflammatory arthritic, infectious, neoplastic, and congenital/developmental pathologies.

As with other uncommon exams, it's useful to have at least a brief background in the anatomy/pathology with teaching videos, or any of the excellent review articles I've referenced. At our institution, we obtain localizers, an axial T2 through the whole head, coronal PD through both TMJs, then sagittal T2 and PD through both TMJs in both closed and open mouth positions. If evaluating for infectious/inflammatory or neoplastic etiologies, postcontrast imaging may also be helpful. Some institutions include dynamic images of the TMJ. What is described here can be generalized to dynamic imaging.

A condensed, step by step approach:

- Check the indication, history, and priors.
  - Remember that you'll likly see the TMJs on any prior CT or MRI study of the head, brain, neck, or cervical spine. Correlating with CT is especially useful to look for calcifications and assess bone morphology.
  - Find out if the patient has any underlying inflammatory arthritic process, or if referring clinicians are concerned about anything other than the usual degenerative TMJ pathology.

- Assess study adequacy.
  - It can be useful to assess the extent that the patient was able to open their mouth. Look for motion or other artifact.

- Look at the localizer images.
  - Evaluate the intracranial compartment, skull base, and upper neck for pathology. As usual, be especially wary of anatomy that is not captured on the other sequences.

- Look at the large FOV axial T2 images.
    - Examine these as you would any usual T2 sequence through the head and brain. At least quickly look at all structures, including the scalp/extracranial soft tissues, bones, sinuses, CSF spaces, and brain parenchyma.
    - Scrutinize the temporal bone mandibular fossa for protrusion of the mandible into the bone.
    - It can useful to hang the sagittal sequences of each joint all together and link them for synchronized scrolling (closed mouth T2, closed mouth PD, open mouth T2, open mouth PD). This allows easy comparison of disc morphology and movement. Comparison of left versus right is also helpful (if you have enough monitor space).

- Look at the T2 images (closed mouth) for soft tissue abnormality:
    - Look for joint effusion.
    - Look for discontinuity of disc attachments posteriorly (retrodiskal tissue rupture).
    - Look for abnormal thickening of disc attachments anteriorly (lateral pterygoid muscle), which may correlate with dysfunction.

      If you see a "double disc" sign (two parallel hypointense bands anterior to the condyle), you might be dealing with an anteriorly displaced disc, seen next to (above) a thickened lateral pterygoid muscle attachment.

- Examine the mandibular condyle (also on T2 images).
    - Look for flattening, osteophytosis, cystic change, and sclerosis.
    - Look for erosions.
    - Look for deformity, as might be seen with inflammatory arthritis or congenital/developmental conditions.
    - Compare morphology with contralateral side as needed.
    - Look for abnormal periarticular signal abnormal, mineral deposition, bone excrescence, or collections/masses.
    - Look at remaining visualized mandible for any other bone lesion, prior fracture, etc.
    - If you can see it, check the mandibular notch for any mass, and mandibular coronoid process for any congenital malformation such as elongation above the level of the zygomatic arch.

    - It can be useful to correlate with any prior CT to look for/characterize osseous abnormalities.

- Assess the PD images (closed mouth) (correlate with T2).
    - Look for normal position of the disc.
        - There should be disc between the mandibular condyle and temporal bone mandibular fossa. Up to 30 degrees anterior displacement from the vertical can be normal.
    - Assess the disc shape/thickness.
        - Normally biconcave, superior side towards the temporal bone mandibular fossa, and the inferior side towards the mandibular condyle.
        - Look for abnormal flattening, discontinuity, or crumpling/irregularity.
    - Assess disc signal.
        - Look for abnormal internal/intrasubstance signal which might reflect perforation/degeneration.

- Assess the T2/PD open mouth views.
    - Assess the degree of mouth opening.
    - Again, look for disc position/translation.
    - The disc should be interposed between the condyle and temporal bone on both open and closed images. The disc should translate slightly anteriorly with the mandibular condyle to the temporal bone articular eminence with mouth opening. If the disc does not move with the condyle, this is abnormal.

- Assess the Coronal PD (closed mouth) views.
    - Assess the medial-lateral position of the disc.
    - Look for displacement.
    - Again, assess disc morphology and signal.
    - Look for degenerative changes at the mandibular condyle.
    - Look for normal relationship between the mandibular condyle and articular fossa, i.e., look for subluxation.

- Repeat the same for the opposite side, comparing left to right as needed.

- Perform some last checks.
    - Look for normal marrow signal in the mandible and skull base.
    - Look for signal abnormality that might suggest a mass lesion or atrophy/denervation of the muscles of mastication.
    - Examine the adjacent teeth and alveolar ridges.
    - Examine the adjacent paranasal sinuses and mastoid air cells.
    - Examine the adjacent parotid gland for masses and other abnormality.
    - Make sure to assess the incidentally imaged neck for masses/adenopathy.
    - Pathology of the surrounding soft tissues and bones can simulate TMJ pathology or extend to and involve the TMJ.
    - If warranted, consider CT to evaluate any bone abnormality.

- Proofread.

References:

1. Tomas X, Pomes J, Berenguer J, Quinto L, Nicolau C, Mercader JM, Castro V. MR imaging of temporomandibular joint dysfunction: a pictorial review. Radiographics. 2006 May;26(3):765-81.
2. Petscavage-Thomas JM, Walker EA. Unlocking the jaw: advanced imaging of the temporomandibular joint. American Journal of Roentgenology. 2014 Nov;203(5):1047-58.

MRI Fetus for CNS Abnormalities

Fetal MRI has been increasingly used to characterize CNS malformations. Ultrasound is often performed first; MRI is used to confirm/exclude suspected pathology, and detect additional abnormality. The development of fast MRI sequences has allowed greater use of these exams, and you may encounter more of these as applications and expertise in the technique grow. Below is an outline of the step-by-step approach we use for this type of study.

- Check the indication, history, and priors.
  - It is essential to know what the clinical question is, even before scanning the patient. You'll want to know if you need to focus the exam on the brain or spine.
  - The exam is generally done after the 18th and preferably the 20th week of gestation. Earlier, and the small size of the fetus with motion artifact can be severely limiting.
  - Many times, fetal MRI will be requested to evaluate a known or questioned abnormality. Having a sense of where this is, and what it could look like will help guide the exam. This will also prime you for potential associated findings. You will almost certainly have prior US, frequently performed by maternal fetal medicine (MFM).
  - Are there prior imaging studies of the mother, including CT/MRI of the abdomen/pelvis? This can help you sort out any incidentally imaged pathology in the mother.
  - Calculate and document the estimated gestational age based on LMP. Look at the most recent US, and reported estimated gestational age based on the US dating as well. This can be the best estimate of gestational age if last LMP is unknown.
  - Gestation age affects the sulcation pattern of brain; it is an essential variable in biometric evaluation. It can be useful to have templates with picklists or reference macros/documents with normal ranges. These can be extracted from the references at the end and/or taken from macros linked in the relevant prior chapter on dictation efficiency.

- Patient preparation.
  - Remove metallic devices/items and jewelry before study.
  - The patient should avoid caffeinated or high-sugar beverages for 4 hours.
  - Assess patient ability to lay decubitus or supine (either is fine). The patient should be able to stay still in the chose position for approximately 45 minutes.
  - Have the patient empty their bladder prior to the study.

- Active exam monitoring and quality assurance.
  - Make sure you have diagnostic quality images in axial, coronal, and sagittal planes through the brain and/or spine, depending on the clinical question.
  - If there is not good signal at the area of concern – brain or spine – ask your technologist to adjust the coil position.
  - If there is persistent motion artifact, and diagnostic quality images cannot be obtained, it is always possible to have the patient return at a later time. This should be done keeping in mind the potential time of any in-utero surgeries/interventions. If the results of fetal MRI are being used to decide on potential termination of pregnancy in the setting of severe/significant pathology, knowledge of local regulations regarding this option is useful in recommending time of follow-up.
  - Note that obtaining diagnostic quality images is at least "half the battle" in fetal MRI.

- Examine the placenta and zygosity.
  - How many fetuses are there?
  - What is the position of the placenta(e)?
    - Where does the umbilical cord insert (if visualized)?
  - Assess the overall volume of amniotic fluid.
  - What is the position of the fetus?
    - Vertex, breech, transverse, or oblique.

- Examine cortical morphology.
  - Assess the sulcation. Look for a normal multilayer appearance of the cortex.
  - Look for any obvious polymicrogyria, lissencepahy (make sure you interpret in context of fetal age), and schizencephaly.

- Look for abnormal migration: subependymal/band heterotopia and subependymal tubers.
- Note however, that you cannot definitively *exclude* migration/formational abnormalities until the myelination process is complete (~2 years old). Therefore, while you can say you don't see anything, it's best to include the caveat that complete evaluation is limited by immaturity of the brain.
- Assess for any destructive processes such as prior infarct or incomplete formation of the cortex.
- Correlate with DWI/ADC maps for infarct.
- Correlate with T1 and SWI for hemorrhage.

- Examine midline structures.
    - Look for presence of the corpus callosum. Make sure you all expected parts, and that they are normal in thickness/formation: the rostrum, genu, body, isthmus, and splenium. A diffusely thinned corpus callosum may represent hypoplasia.
    - Look for the normal cavum septum pellucidum. Absence is correlated with other midline abnormalities such as callosal dysgenesis/agenesis. This can help improve diagnostic certainty, as the corpus callosum is often difficult to visualize well if there are study limitations from motion or other artifact.
    - Examine the optic chiasm, pituitary, and infundibulum, up to limitation of technique.
    - Look for normal separation of the cerebral hemispheres: look at the medial frontal lobes, thalami, and posterior falx (for the spectrum of holoprosencephaly). Correlate with any facial abnormalities.

- Examine the posterior fossa.
    - Look for small/malformed cerebellar hemispheres, vermis, and/or brainstem. Look for a "molar tooth" sign, as seen in Joubert syndrome.
    - Compare vermis size to normal measurement of age for possible vermian hypoplasia (Dandy walker variant).
    - Look for Dandy-Walker spectrum abnormalities, including posterior fossa cyst and vermian hypoplasia.

  - Measure the tegmentovermian angle, which helps differentiate between the various Dandy-Walker spectrum abnormalities.
  - Look for abnormal crowding of the posterior fossa and tonsillar ectopia, as seen in Chiari malformations.

- Examine the ventricular system.
  - Look for hydrocephalus, e.g., ventricular atrial enlargement >10 mm. Consider within context of overall brain/cranial size.
  - Look for parallel orientation of the ventricular system and colpocephaly, as seen with callosal abnormalities.

- Examine the entire spine.
  - Use all available planes, though sagittal and axials will likely be most useful.
  - Look for abnormal formation/segmentation anomalies.
  - Look for dysraphic abnormalities, including iniencephaly, cephalocele, meningocele, myelomeningocele.
  - Look for spinal and para spinal masses.

- Examine the face/neck soft tissues, as warranted/prompted by neurologic findings.
  - Look for absent, small, or abnormally spaced eyes.
  - Look for absent or malformed nasal bridge.
  - Look for choanal atresia.
  - Look for cleft lip/palate, maxillary or mandibular hypoplasia.
  - Look for teeth abnormalities, so such single midline molar.
  - Look for lateral facial clefts, ear malformations and clefts.
  - Look for calvarial deformities.
  - Look for any obvious mass lesions and lymphatic/vascular malformations.

- Measure and compare the following to normal biometric ranges (based on gestational age/in references).
  - Right ventricle atrium.
  - Left ventricle atrium.
  - Length of the corpus callosum.
  - Cerebral biparietal diameter.
  - Bone biparietal diameter.
  - Vermis AP diameter.

    - Vermis height.
    - Cerebellum coronal diameter.
    - Pons AP diameter.
    - *Note:* quantitative assessment can help you detect subtle abnormality better than visual inspection. Whether or not you report values in the dictation is up to institutional/personal preference.

- The non-neurological structures may be examined and reported by a pediatric radiologist.
    - Document their name and findings. They will look for gross abnormalities of the chest, abdomen, pelvis, limbs, and placenta.
    - Remember to document that the exam is not tailored to these structures.
    - In some institutions, you may look at these yourself and only consult a pediatric radiologist if there is gross abnormality/as needed. A full discussion of this process is outside the scope of this text. Two references below (Saleem & Manganaro) provide an orientation if needed.

- It can be useful to look at incidentally imaged maternal abdominopelvic anatomy, for the rare case of maternal pathology you'll see.

- Proofread and discuss the finding with the referring services as warranted.

References:

1. Saleem SN. Fetal MRI: An approach to practice: A review. Journal of advanced research. 2014 Sep 1;5(5):507-23.
2. Manganaro L, Antonelli A, Bernardo S, Capozza F, Petrillo R, Satta S, Vinci V, Saldari M, Maccioni F, Ballesio L, Catalano C. Highlights on MRI of the fetal body. La radiologia medica. 2018 Apr;123(4):271-85.
3. Masselli G, Notte MV, Zacharzewska-Gondek A, Laghi F, Manganaro L, Brunelli R. Fetal MRI of CNS abnormalities. Clinical radiology. 2020 Apr 26.
4. Nagarajan M, Sharbidre KG, Bhabad SH, Byrd SE. MR imaging of the fetal face: comprehensive review. RadioGraphics. 2018 May;38(3):962-80.
5. Parazzini C, Righini A, Rustico M, Consonni D, Triulzi F. Prenatal magnetic resonance imaging: brain normal linear biometric values below 24 gestational weeks. Neuroradiology. 2008 Oct 1;50(10):877-83.
6. Tilea B, Alberti C, Adamsbaum C, Armoogum P, Oury JF, Cabrol D, Sebag G, Kalifa G, Garel C. Cerebral biometry in fetal magnetic resonance imaging: new reference data. Ultrasound in Obstetrics and Gynecology. 2009 Feb;33(2):173-81.

Search Patterns for Uncommon CT Studies

Long H. Tu

Amit Mahajan

Ichiro Ikuta

4D CT for Parathyroid Adenomas

The "4D" CT for parathyroid adenomas makes use of multiphase contrast enhanced CT to help localize suspected abnormal parathyroid glands. It's important to note that it is *not* used to diagnose primary hyperparathyroidism. Existing biochemical diagnosis is a prerequisite for doing such a study, and should be done prior to approval of the 4D CT.

The classic appearance of a parathyroid adenoma is an oval, arterially enhancing lesion, which may be associated with a polar feeding vessel. Some parathyroid adenomas may be best detected on the delayed images (faster wash out than thyroid) or non-contrast (lower attenuation than thyroid). You will need to do a dedicated search on each phase of contrast. Adenomas may also have cystic foci, fatty components or calcification. Because the purpose of the study is to identify all potential lesions which may be adenomas, it is worthwhile to suspect all soft tissue nodules which cannot be confidently excluded as blood vessel, lymph node, or thyroid nodule.

One useful approach is to look first at the eutopic locations, then likely ectopic locations, in each of the arterial, delayed, and pre-contrast image sets. It can be useful to hang all the axial images together, and all the coronal/sagittal images together (of differing phases), to correlate across different projections. Make sure to keep looking, even if you find an obvious/likely adenoma, as a significant minority of patients will have multiglandular disease. Then systematically evaluate the remainder of the study for incidental findings. Report every candidate lesion, with level of confidence, size, and location relative to surgical landmarks. Below is a suggested approach.

- Check the indication, history, and priors.
    - Get a sense as to the level of clinical suspicion/confidence that the patient has primary hyperparathyroidism.
    - Make sure to look at prior ultrasound, MRI, and/or scintigraphic studies that may have clues as to where you might find an adenoma.
    - Note any prior studies covering the same neck/chest anatomy prior to the development of hyperparathyroidism. Nodules that have characteristic features and are new/increased compared to these priors are more suspicious for adenoma. A long-standing nodule that has not changed

from a remote timepoint to the time of hyperparathyroidism onset is less suspicious.

- On the arterial phase images:
  - Look for avidly enhancing lesions (greater than thyroid).
    - Look for any characteristic polar feeding vessels.
  - Search at eutopic locations:
    - Around the thyroid, both anterior and posterior to the tracheoesophageal groove. Most commonly, you'll see adenomas just posterior or just inferior to the thyroid gland.
    - Adenomas may be difficult to differentiate from normal thyroid tissue or exophytic nodules. Use multiple planes of imaging, and look closely at differential enhancement (across phases).
    - Don't forget the thyroid gland can have a normal variant, a tubercle of Zuckerkandl. It can look like a nodule if you are not paying close attention. It is also a useful anatomic landmark for surgeons since the recurrent laryngeal nerve is expected to be medial to it.
  - Search at ectopic locations:
    - Look at the retropharyngeal and retroesophageal spaces, in the carotid sheath, in the scalene fat pad. Look *within* the thyroid gland, all the spaces between the thyroid and thymus (thyrothymic ligament), and *within* the thymus. Look within the visualized mediastinum.
    - Intrathyroid parathyroid adenomas, although rare and thyroid nodules can have a similar appearance on 4D CT images. These can be differentiated by other modalities (ultrasound, MRI, nuclear medicine) as warranted.
    - Very rarely, parathyroid adenomas can be found in unusual locations such as the posterior triangle of the neck, axilla, pericardium, and others. If you cannot localize an adenoma in the more common

ectopic locations, keep looking/keep an eye out when assessing the remainder of the study.

- Assess all the above spaces in at least two planes, ideally axial and coronal.
- Remember to keep looking even if you've found one or more likely/candidate lesions, as 10% of patients will have multiglandular disease. Note that you may see mild enlargement of multiple small (often eutopic) glands. In this case, consider the possibility of parathyroid hyperplasia – an uncommon cause of primary hyperparathyroidism.

- On the delayed images:
    - Look for lesions that wash out more than thyroid. Some adenomas are only well visualized on delayed images, as the contrast from the surrounding vessels fades away.
    - Search the eutopic and ectopic locations systematically, as above.

- On non-contrast images:
    - Look for lesions that are lower attenuation than thyroid. Some adenomas are only well visualized on non-contrast images.
    - Search the eutopic and ectopic locations systematically, as above.

- Look at the rest of the study.
    - It can be useful to do a usual CT neck search pattern through the delayed (close to venous/parenchymal phase) images.
        - Compare with the non-contrast to assess enhancement versus inherent hyperdensity.
        - Use the arterial phase images to assess the neck arterial vasculature.
        - Do not forget to look at *everything:* the neck nodal distribution, aerodigestive tract/mucosal surfaces, exocrine glands, vessels, bones, brain, lungs, mediastinum, soft tissues. We have seen incidental lung cancers, cervical adenopathy, breast masses, etc.

  - Make sure that if the patient moved in between phases that you look at the edges of the image set for each phase. You may see additional lung parenchyma or face/brain anatomy on different phases.

- Report each candidate adenoma.
  - Report the total number of candidate adenomas.
  - Report size (greatest dimension) of each.
  - Report location relative to surgical landmarks (cricoid cartilage, tracheoesophageal groove, thyroid gland, and suprasternal notch).
  - Report your level of confidence that the nodule represents an adenoma.
  - Comment on concurrent thyroid abnormalities/nodules, which may require work up or promote concurrent resection.
  - Remember to compare to any prior studies (including other modalities) where the same anatomic sites may have been imaged.

- Report other/incidental findings
  - Aortic arch anomalies, e.g., aberrant right subclavian artery. These impact surgical approach (related to non-recurrent laryngeal nerve).
  - Other incidentals discovered during systematic search through the anatomy.

- Proofread.

References:

1. Hoang JK, Sung WK, Bahl M, Phillips CD. How to perform parathyroid 4D CT: tips and traps for technique and interpretation. Radiology. 2014 Jan;270(1):15-24.
2. Bunch PM, Randolph GW, Brooks JA, George V, Cannon J, Kelly HR. Parathyroid 4D CT: What the Surgeon Wants to Know. RadioGraphics. 2020 Sep;40(5):1383-94.
3. Murphy A, Deng F, et al. Parathyroid 4D CT. https://radiopaedia.org/articles/parathyroid-4d-ct?lang=us. Accessed 6/21/2021.
4. Chang BA, Sharma A, Anderson DW. Ectopic parathyroid adenoma in the soft palate: a case report. Journal of Otolaryngology-Head & Neck Surgery. 2016 Dec;45(1):1-4.

CT Conebeam Maxillofacial Notes

At our institution, we do conebeam CT exams for the presurgical evaluation of maxillofacial abnormalities as well as to follow post-operative changes. In most cases, the images are obtained for plastic surgeons or oromaxillofacial surgeons to visualize the bony anatomy, and the formal radiologic evaluation seldom alters clinical management. The areas where we make a difference are in finding unexpected underlying osseous lesions, anatomic variants, and in systematically evaluating for hardware failure or other unexpected post-operative complication.

Many of the terms and concepts used in the surgical planning may be unfamiliar to new fellows. If CT conebeam exams are part of your practice/fellowship, I highly recommend the Medscape review article on orthognathic ("jaw correction") surgery referenced at the end of this chapter for a deeper discussion. It will key you into almost every concept you'll need to know to understand what is happening with these patients. Without a deeper familiarity, you can still get some degree of orientation by reading the clinical notes for any individual case (always a good practice).

In this section, I'll first provide a set of essential concepts used in orthognathic surgery pulled from the references, with translation into similar radiographic terminology. Many of these are not covered in usual neuroradiology texts. While not always necessary for interpreting studies, understanding these will give you a sense as to what the surgery will "correct." Subsequently, I'll describe the brief checklist I keep in mind when looking at these studies. I'll assume you already have an approach to conventional CT head/facial bone studies.

Dental Terms Explained –Anatomic Surfaces/Directions of Teeth

- Distal – Surface Away from the midline of the face.
- Mesial – Surface that is closest to the midline of the face.
- Facial – Surface that faces the cheeks or lips.
    a. Labial – Surface towards the lips.
    b. Buccal – Surface towards the cheeks.
- Lingual –Surface that faces the tongue.
- Incisal – Biting edge of an anterior tooth.
- Occlusal – Chewing surface of posterior teeth.
- Proximal – Tooth surfaces that are next to each other (i.e., distal surface of lateral incisor and mesial surface of canine).

Orthognathic Terms Explained

- Overjet - *Horizontal* distance between the incisal edges of the maxillary incisor to the mandibular incisor (i.e., how far apart are the front teeth in the AP direction?).
- Overbite - *Vertical* distance between the incisal edge of the maxillary incisor and the mandibular incisor (i.e., how far apart are the front teeth in the craniocaudal (CC) direction?).
- Crossbite - Lingual-buccal malposition of the normal relationship between the upper and lower dentition (i.e., do the teeth line up in the transverse (TV) direction?).
- Deep bite - Condition of excessive overbite (front teeth overlap in CC direction).
- Open bite - Condition of negative overbite (front teeth do not meet in CC direction, producing a gap).
- Retrognathism – Relatively *posterior* position (of the mandible or maxilla) to the skeletal base. This is assessed relative to line in the coronal plane of the skull.
- Prognathism – Relatively anterior position/protrusion (of the mandible or maxilla) to the skeletal base. This is assessed relative to line in the coronal plane of the skull.

Orthognathic Surgical Procedures and their Usual Indications

- Le Fort I osteotomy – Used to correct maxillary deficiency or excess.
- Le Fort II osteotomy - Used to correct midface hypoplasia involving the maxilla and nasal complex.
- Le Fort III osteotomy - Used to correct midface hypoplasia involving the nasal, maxillary, and orbital/zygomatic complexes.
- Bilateral sagittal split osteotomies (BSSO) – Corrects mandibular prognathia or retrognathia.
- Genioplasty – Corrects chin excess/deficiency (often cosmetic)
- "Triple jaw surgery" – Refers to combination of three procedures: Le Fort I + BSSO + genioplasty.
- Note: some patients will have personalized/tailored surgeries based on specific needs, that use combinations of the above elements and other components/fixation.

Malocclusion Classifications

There are two common means of classifying malocclusion (when teeth are misaligned with a closed mouth). One depends on the relationship of the first molars, and the other depends on the relationship of the incisors.

Molar Classification of Malocclusion (Angle Classification)

- Class I – The position of the dental arches is normal, with first molars in normal occlusion.
- Class II – The relationship of the dental arches is abnormal, with all the mandibular teeth occluding distal to normal.
  - Class II division 1 – The maxillary incisors are protruding labially;
  - Class II division 2 – The maxillary incisors are lingually inclined.
- Class III – The relationship of the dental arches is abnormal, with all mandibular teeth occluding mesial to normal.

Incisor Classification of Malocclusion

- Class I – The mandibular incisor tips occlude or lie below the cingulum plateau of the maxillary incisors.
- Class II – The mandibular incisor tips occlude or lie posterior to the cingulum plateau (the concave, lingual aspect of the tooth adjacent to the incisive surface) of the maxillary incisors. This classification is further subdivided into:
    - Class II division 1 – The overjet is increased with upright or proclined (pointed anterior) maxillary incisors.
    - Class II division 2 – The maxillary incisors are retroclined (pointed posterior), with a normal or occasionally increased overjet.
- Class III – The mandibular incisor tips occlude or lie anterior to the cingulum plateau of the maxillary incisors.

Suggested Checklist for Assessment

- Check the indication, history, and prior studies.
    - Note that any prior conventional CT/MRI studies may better delineate abnormities than conebeam CT.
    - Have a sense as to any underlying syndrome, prior trauma, or prior surgery.
    - Having a sense as to what surgery (if any) is being planned, and what orthognathic/maxillofacial abnormalities are being addressed can help prime you to understand the anatomy and what to expect post-operatively.
    - Some patients will also have a presenting symptom/complaint outside of surgical planning. Knowing what this is can help you look for incidental explanatory pathologies.

- Assess the osseous structures in usual fashion.
    - Look specifically for lucent/sclerotic osseous lesions.
    - Look for deformity and prior/healing fractures.
    - Look at the temporomandibular joints (TMJ) to see if they are intact.

    - Check the mandibular coronoid processes for hyperplasia (extension higher than the zygomatic arches).
    - Check the paranasal sinuses and mastoid air cells for opacification/unexpected pathology. These are often opacified in the immediate post-operative state.
    - Look for incidental dental pathology, e.g., periapical lucencies/periodontal disease and caries. Periodontal disease may warrant referral if not already known.

- Assess the soft tissues to the extent able.
    - You'll generally only be able to see large/obvious pathology, as conebeam CT does not resolve soft tissues as clearly as conventional CT. We include a caveat in our dictations that the soft tissues are not well evaluated using conebeam CT technique.
    - Look at the orbits and face soft tissues for obvious mass lesion/collection, adenopathy, and inflammatory changes. Even evaluating the skin surface for asymmetry may be useful.

- For post-surgical studies:
    - Look for usual signs of hardware failure: hardware fracture, displacement/malposition, and periprosthetic fracture. Make sure to look at *all* the bones, as unexpected or new fractures may be seen in sites somewhat removed from the surgery.
    - Be sure to look for new TMJ malalignment/dislocation.
    - If the patient had prior fractures/dislocations, make sure you describe which of these have been addressed, and which remain. Note any change in alignment.
    - For immediate post-op, if the intracranial compartment has been entered or involved (often due to underling bony abnormality), assess extent of pneumocephalus and consider any sites that might be culprits should the patient have concern for CSF leak. Look for collections/hematomas.

- Proofread.

References:

1. Orthognathic Surgery https://emedicine.medscape.com/article/1279747-overview#showall Accessed: 5/15/2021.
2. Foster VP. An Overview of Dental Anatomy. https://www.dentalcare.com/en-us/professional-education/ce-courses/ce500/surfaces-of-the-teeth Accessed: 5/15/2021.

Dual Energy CT Head

A common use of dual energy CT head is differentiating iodine/contrast staining and hemorrhage. Other indications include to assess the extent of iodine leak (active extravasation) in acute intracranial hemorrhage, use of bone/calcium subtraction to improve characterization of arterial pathology or detection of subtle extra-axial blood, and virtual monochromatic imaging for metal artifact reduction. I'll focus on the first of these – differentiating iodine and blood, as this is likely the first that a fellow will encounter.

At our institution, we are provided the dual energy virtual monochromatic images (VMI, "mixed energy"), an iodine map, virtual non-contrast (VNC) images, and virtual non-calcium (VNCa) images. Make sure that you can clearly identify which of these is which, as the VNC and VMI can appear very similar. The approach is straightforward once you're oriented to which image is which. Below is the organization I use – an already familiar approach to conventional CT head imaging is assumed.

- Check the indication, history, and priors.
    - Know any prior stroke territory. Look at any prior conventional CT/MRI head. Know if the patient has received intra-arterial contrast or other contrast enhanced studies (CTA head and neck, digital subtraction cerebral angiogram, etc.)

- Assess the mixed energy images as you would any usual head CT.
    - Note any areas of hyperdensity that the other images will help you differentiate into different materials.

- Assess the VNC images.
    - Compare these to the mixed energy images. Any hyperdensity still seen on the VNC is likely blood (rarely, calcium). As with conventional CT, narrow windows can help you detect subtle abnormality.
    - Note that for suspected areas of hemorrhage, you can have adjacent or mixed iodine AND blood. The hyperdensity may get smaller or less dense on the VNC compared to the mixed energy images. What remains is the area of true blood product (contrast/iodine has been removed). Remember that

remaining blood products can be isodense if it is hyperacute, subacute, and/or the patient is severely anemic.

- Assess the iodine map.
    - These images can also be windowed. It is essential to use narrow windows to make areas of subtle iodine as conspicuous as possible.
    - Correlate the iodine distribution with the areas of hyperdensity that were "missing" on the VNC. The VNC and iodine map should "add up" to the mixed images.
    - If the dual energy CT head is done without concurrent IV contrast, areas on the iodine map would represent contrast staining. If concurrent IV contrast is administered, consider that concentrated iodine within hematomas could represent active extravasation ("spot sign"). This is the same phenomenon as a "swirl sign" on non-contrast CT head in the setting of active bleeding.
    - The iodine map can also be used to assess degree of enhancement with any inherently dense mass, though this will be a less common scenario.
    - Often times the iodine map will have a colored hue (for example, our institution has iodine appear with increased orange hue). These colors may vary by vendor, and can be customized via the image post-processing software package.
    - Because color detection is important, make sure you are inspecting the iodine map on a color monitor (not a strictly black-and-white monitor). Also consider a clinical validation test case for any radiologists that might be color blind when setting the iodine map color.

- Assess the virtual non-calcium (VNCa) images.
    - One use of VNCa images for any dual energy CT head would be to distinguish calcium from hemorrhage. Especially if there are no prior exams for comparison and if the hyperattenuation is punctate (so almost no edema would be seen), the VNCa can be very useful.

        - If the mixed energy images show a punctate hyperdensity, and it is not seen on the VNCa, then it is calcium.
        - If the mixed energy images show a punctate hyperdensity, and it persists on the VNCa, then you need to be concerned for hemorrhage (petechial or subarachnoid).
    - VNCa images are useful to check the cerebral convexities and areas near the skull base for subtle extra-axial blood/masses. Subtraction of adjacent bone can make these more conspicuous.
    - Compared to conventional CTA, "bone subtraction" CTA can be more sensitive to stenosis adjacent to calcification or at the skull base. However, stenosis tends to be *overestimated*, due to subtraction of blooming. A reasonable approach would be to use bone subtraction to detect vessel lesions, and rely on the mixed energy images to characterize any stenosis. (Accuracy for other vascular lesions is comparable, and bone subtracted vessel assessment can be faster).

- Make sure to compare any findings to prior.

- Proofread.

References:

1. Potter CA, Sodickson AD. Dual-energy CT in emergency neuroimaging: added value and novel applications. Radiographics. 2016 Nov;36(7):2186-98.
2. Postma AA, Das M, Stadler AA, Wildberger JE. Dual-energy CT: what the neuroradiologist should know. Current radiology reports. 2015 May;3(5):1-6.

Checklists for Advanced MRI Studies

Long H. Tu

Mariam Aboian

Ichiro Ikuta

Functional MRI (fMRI)

Functional MRI is most often performed at our institution for presurgical planning prior to resection of an epileptogenic focus or tumor. Vital to fMRI are isotropic imaging with 3D FLAIR or 3D T1 images to allow for adequate spatial resolution. Since our institution also co-registers the pre-surgical fMRI with the intra-operative MRI in the operating room, we specially protocol the isotropic images to include the tip of the nose, back of the head, top of the head/vertex, and the ears. No headphones or video goggles should be worn, as these distort the surface anatomy, although special lenses/mirrors are used to allow the patient to see the screen located just outside of the MRI bore. Depending upon the indication, IV contrast may or may not be needed.

The most important objective is to lateralize language function and to map essential areas of motor function relative to the lesion. We perform DTI tractography to assist with planning of resection relative to major white matter pathways.

Differing institutions will perform different tasks for mapping. We always do a verbal assessment (word generation, verb generation, and sentence completion), and sometimes object naming for patients with reduced mental capacity. Motor tasks depend upon lesion location, most commonly we do upper extremity motor task (finger tapping). Lower extremity movement (foot tapping) or facial motor (lip movement) can be done in special circumstances. We use a task reference book to prepare patients for the study that summarizes all the actions they need to take.

All our fMRIs are actively monitored by a fellow and/or attending. This quality control allows you to see if the patient is actually following directions, allowing you to make adjustments to tasks if needed. Being present for the critical portions of the exam also allows you to troubleshoot any issues as they arise. Below is a checklist modeled after our institutional workflow. Most items will apply to fMRI workflow at any institution.

- Review the indication, history, and prior imaging.
    - Know the lesion in question, especially if there are multiple brain abnormalities.
    - Review the patient's history in the electronic medical record and prior brain imaging. If a lesion/tumor is known to enhance, then an IV will need to be started. If planning for

resection of a seizure focus that does not enhance, no IV is necessary.
  - Know what language the patient speaks/reads.

- Meet the patient (and any family). This is your opportunity to explain the study and maximize the chance that the patient will be able to cooperate to the best of their ability.
  - Consider a script such as: "If you have had an MRI scan before, this will be similar. The only difference is that for part of the scan we will give you tasks to perform so that we can see what part of your brain you use to do different things. Don't worry about remembering these instructions. When it's time to do a task, we will go over the instructions again to make sure you are ready. This is not a graded test, just relax and do the best you can."
  - Go through the fMRI "educational manual," explaining each of the tasks with the patient. Make sure to obtain one matching the patient's preferred language. Use an interpreter when needed when speaking with the patient prior to the exam. Our institution also uses software that provides directions and language tasks in several languages; check with your vendor for options. It is important to get the patient to relax, as this can improve the chance that they will complete the entire exam. As much as possible, express confidence, reassurance, and a willingness to help if asked.
  - This is a good time to get a sense of the patient's ability to cooperate with the study. Some patients, whether due to the lesion in question or other underlying conditions, may not be able to follow commands. This will help prime you to how much real-time coaching you will have to do, and to what extent you will be able to believe the results of the study.
  - See if the patient can read and do the required movements (e.g., finger tapping). If an anatomic region is paralyzed, you can alternatively go into the MRI scanner room and rub the patient's fingers/toes (1st web space) with gauze or passively move the patient's finger/toe to generate a signal. As usual, make sure you do not have any ferromagnetic items on your person and are otherwise are able to enter an MRI Zone 4.

  - Check if the patient will need glasses to read the screen. They cannot bring their own glasses into the MR scanner. At our institution, the technologist staff keep MR safe glasses, which are available on request.
  - Once all the patient's and family's questions are answered, let the technologists know that patient is ready. They will prepare and position the patient in the scanner.

- For hand or foot movement tasks, consider the scripts such as the following to coach the patient, and optimize the study.
  - "Can you see the hands (or cross) okay?"
  - "When the picture of the hand (or foot) appears, start tapping your thumb to index finger (or tap your big toe), and keep tapping as long as the picture is flashing."
  - "Keep the rest of your body still during the study, move only your right/left hand/foot."
  - Watch the patients to confirm that movement/task is performed correctly. It should start on cue, and stop when the stimulus/prompt stops. The hand (or foot) should more smoothly. The patient should not lift the arm or leg, or move other parts of their body. They should also not be speaking. These other movements will produce off-target signal.
  - For all tasks, provide both reassurance and reminders. Consider "You're doing a great job!" and "Remember to keep your head/body as still as possible."

- For verbal tasks, consider the following scripts for coaching.
  - "Are you able to see the words?"
  - For a sentence completion task: "Read the sentence to yourself and fill in the word that makes the most sense. Remember not to say the words out loud or move your mouth. Just think of the words in your mind. Repeat the sentence in your head if it is still there."

  - For cues that are used to obtain background activity, you can coach the patient with a script such as: "When you see (no instructions) you can just look at the screen and relax – try to let your mind go blank."

- Preparation of the scanner and patient.
  - Make sure the MRI technologists know to include the patient's nose, ears, back of the head, and top of the head in the images. These are areas necessary for co-registration for intra-operative image guidance. If these areas are outside of the field of view, ask the MRI techs to include necessary areas in a repeat sequence.
  - On our system, the DTI images must be obtained in as close to true axial as possible. No head tilting or obliquity of image acquisition is allowed.

  - In performing fMRI for seizures, ask the technologists for the following sequences:
    - 3D T1 pre-contrast (MPRAGE).
    - Word generation (BOLD).
    - Verb generation (BOLD).
    - Sentence completion (BOLD).
    - Right finger tapping (BOLD).
    - Left finger tapping (BOLD).
    - Repeat any tasks as needed, if poor signal.
    - DTI – no head tilt, straight axial.
    - 3D FLAIR.
    - Coronal T2 from institutional seizure protocol.
    - Rest of the protocol, including sagittal/coronal. reformats of MPRAGE and FLAIR sequences.
    - Lesion specific imaging (such as SWI for blood or calcification).
  - In performing fMRI for tumor or other enhancing lesions, ask for the following sequences. Structural imaging is obtained first, so that in case the patient is unable to continue with the study, the neurosurgeons will at least have an anatomic orientation.
    - Localizers.

    - Pre-contrast 3D T1 (MPRAGE).
    - Perfusion if ordered.
    - Post-contrast 3D T1 (MPRAGE 3D T1 Post).
    - DTI – no head tilt, straight axial.
    - Word generation (BOLD).
    - Verb generation (BOLD).
    - Sentence completion (BOLD).
    - Right finger tapping (BOLD).
    - Left finger tapping (BOLD).
    - Repeat any tasks as needed, if poor signal.
    - 3D FLAIR.
    - Rest of the protocol, including sagittal/coronal reformats of MPRAGE and FLAIR sequences.

- Since fMRI is not as commonly performed as other exams, it may be helpful to write down the tasks you would like performed, any special/extra sequences, and then provide it to the MRI technologist so everyone is on the same page.

- Watch the beginning of the study and make sure early/structural sequences are of sufficient quality to delineate the lesion from normal (or relatively normal) brain tissue.

- Perform real time quality assurance.
    - As the images for each task are obtained, look to see if there is sufficient signal to noise to localize activation. Note that especially for patients with large lesions or significant underlying pathology, the pattern of activation can be reorganized, bilateral, or distorted compared to expected regions in normal patients.
    - If the signal to noise is not acceptable for any verbal or motor tasks, consider repeating that task. Be especially care to coach the patient and watch for deviations from the task with the repeat images.

- Confirm transfer of images to required PACS.
    - Not all technologists may be familiar with the fMRI workflow. Make sure that they send the images to both your

post-processing server as well as any operating room system if surgical teams use the images for real-time localization.

- Postprocess the fMRI BOLD data.
  - Different institutions will have differing software packages for postprocessing. The major steps are outlined below to provide a sense the overall logic.
  - Display the anatomic images (FLAIR or T1 post-contrast) and overlay the BOLD data from the first of your fMRI paradigms.
  - Check that there is ideally less than 1 degree of rotation/motion. More than this, and you may not be able to trust that your task-specific activity registers appropriately to expected brain anatomy.
  - Using a qualitative/overall assessment of expected brain activation for each task (as corresponds to the appropriate Brodman/brain-homunculus site), chose a balance of signal to noise that highlights the likely site of activation for the task in question. This ideally maintains $p<0.05$, and an overall negative activation of <10%, as qualitatively assessed when looking at the brain volume.
  - If you do not see any activation at the $p=0.05$ threshold, consider increasing the sensitivity/signal above the 0.05 level to see if you can delineate an area of activation. Note that you should report that this signal was NOT statistically significant using whichever metric is employed by your software/workflow.
  - Repeat post-processing for every paradigm.
  - If image tasks are color-coded, remember which is which (take notes), so that you can provide guidance in your dictation.

- Postprocess the DTI raw data.
  - For most fMRI studies, you will want to visualize the "tracts" of at least the arcuate fasciculus (for language) and corticospinal tracts for sensorimotor evaluation.
  - Select the arcuate fasciculus using a coronal view of the DTI images between the expected location of the Broca's area

  - and Wernicke's area. Selecting green (anteroposterior) tracts are usually the most useful. It is useful to do this bilaterally.
  - Select the corticospinal tracts using a region of interest on axial images in the pons, or if needed at the posterior limb of the internal capsule or at the cerebral peduncles.
  - Additional fibers can be added if there is sparse "seeding" and errant fibers can be subtracted using software tools.

- Overlay, label, and send the data to PACS.
  - Overlaying all of the language tasks improves accuracy of localizing language function in the brain. Include the arcuate fasciculus/superior longitudinal fasciculus tracts bilaterally (but not the sensorimotor activations/tracts).
  - Send axial, coronal, and sagittal reformats of the language tasks/tracts (all overlaid) to PACS and the OR.
  - Separately, do the same for sensorimotor tasks and corticospinal tracts (blue on DTI), in all 3 planes, and send to PACS and the OR.

- Report the study.
  - Interpret the conventional MRI sequences as usual.
  - Provide a key as to the color scheme of each fMRI task.
  - Comment on distance between the center of task activation and the leading edge of a lesion.
  - Comment on lesion distance or involvement of the major white major tracts. Include measurements from the lesion periphery to the periphery of the white matter tracts.
  - Note lateralization of language (left, right, mixed, co-dominant). Areas of task overlap increase confidence of language localization. If unclear, recommendation could be made for WADA test and/or psychological testing.
  - Remember to interpret within the context of any technical or patient cooperation limitations. If these are sufficient to degrade confidence in task localization, the neurosurgeons may be able to do intraoperative direct cortical stimulation.

- Remember to proofread.

References:

1. Silva MA, See AP, Essayed WI, Golby AJ, Tie Y. Challenges and techniques for presurgical brain mapping with functional MRI. NeuroImage: Clinical. 2018 Jan 1;17:794-803.
2. Black DF, Vachha B, Mian A, Faro SH, Maheshwari M, Sair HI, Petrella JR, Pillai JJ, Welker K. American Society of Functional Neuroradiology-Recommended fMRI Paradigm Algorithms for Presurgical Language Assessment. AJNR Am J Neuroradiol. 2017 Oct;38(10):E65-E73. doi: 10.3174/ajnr.A5345. Epub 2017 Aug 31. PMID: 28860215; PMCID: PMC7963630.

MR Spectroscopy (MRS)

The most common indications we encounter for MRS are characterization of an indeterminate brain lesion and to help predict grade of a glioma. It is essential to verify the patient history and study appropriateness, as at the time of this writing, many indications may not be covered by insurance. Below is a brief checklist on screening, consulting on, and performing these uncommon studies.

- Check the indication, history, and look at any priors.
    - Check specifically notes written by the requesting physician/provider, as they will often explain the underlying reasoning. Check to see what lesion is being characterized and what the suspected underlying etiologies are.
    - Check to see that prior MRI and possibly MR perfusion studies have been performed. MRS and MR perfusion are complementary and both together have increased accuracy.
    - Make sure the indication fits one of the usual/appropriate uses of MRS:
        - Distinguishing low grade from high grade gliomas (complementary to structural MRI and MR perfusion).
        - Characterization of an indeterminate brain lesion for planning or deferral of biopsy/resection.
        - Distinguishing recurrent brain tumor from radiation-induced tumor necrosis (complementary to structural MRI and MR perfusion).
        - Pediatric disorders including hypoxic ischemic encephalopathy, inherited neurometabolic diseases, and traumatic brain injury.
        - In rare cases, MRS can be used to help differentiate infection (including fungal etiologies) from other processes.
    - If the indication/history or other details do not make sense, contact the referring clinician/team to get more details. Knowing exactly what you're looking for is essential to performing this study correctly.

- Note the patient age, as patients of varying age (especially neonates and the elderly) may have baseline spectra that vary from normal adults.

- Chose acquisition parameters.
    - Chose multivoxel imaging to characterize large/heterogeneous lesion, multifocal processes, and for regional metabolic variations. This covers most scenarios.
    - Single voxel imaging is sometimes used for a smaller lesion or diffuse process, to improve signal to noise, or when multivoxel technique is not available.
    - You'll also need a spectrum at a contralateral (normal) area of brain for comparison for both multivoxel and single voxel analyses.
    - Using both medium and long TE (e.g., 135ms and 270ms) allows differentiation of the lactate peak, which is inverted in medium TEs. Longer TE improves visualization of Cho, Cr, and NAA peaks by suppressing metabolites with short T2 values (e.g., lipids, glutamate, glutamine, GABA, glucose, and myo-inositol).
    - Place the volume of interest.
        - Include the lesion based on the MR structural images.
        - For the voxel used to characterize an abnormality, *exclude* normal brain, CSF, and bone/scalp. Avoid susceptibility artifact. This mitigates against volume averaging effects and erroneous signal. Make sure there are voxels at each of the sites of any lesion heterogeneity that you are looking to characterize. Minimize any areas of central necrosis (you already know it is necrosis, but the periphery could be viable tumor, and that is the clinical question).
        - In single voxel MRS, use a second voxel at the contralateral brain to assess normal brain signal. Similarly, exclude CSF, bone/scalp, and any susceptibility artifact.

- Examine the MRS spectrum. Assess presence/overall peak magnitude of the following components:
    - N- Acetylaspartate (NAA) - 2 ppm.
    - Choline - 3.2 ppm.
    - Lactate - 1.3 ppm (inverted on intermediate TE).
    - Lipid/macromolecules - 1.3 ppm.
    - Myo-inositol - 3.5 ppm.

- In rare cases of evaluation for potential infectious etiology, look for the following peaks:
    - Amino acids (valine leucine and isoleucine) - 0.9.
    - Lipid/lactate (Lip/lac) - 0.9 to 1.4, 1.3.
    - Alanine - 1.46.
    - Acetate - 1.92.
    - Succinate - 2.4.
    - Glycine 3.56.
    - Trehalose 3.6 to 3.8 (specific for fungal infections).

- What is the overall concentration/level of metabolites?
    - Overall decreases, e.g., in subacute stroke can simulate disease.
    - Remember to rescale/normalize the y-axis when comparing differing plots.
    - Assess the Hunter's angle.
    - What is the Choline to NAA ratio? Higher ratios (>2.0-2.5) predict high grade tumor. Lower ratios predict low grade tumor or non-neoplastic processes.

- Notes on interpretation:
    - A full discussion of MRS limitations, sensitivity, and interpretation is outside of the scope of this process-focused section. However, a few points can be helpful to keep in mind. The below curated set of notes should be enough for most practical purposes.

- Tumor:
  - High grade gliomas: higher Chol/NAA ratio (>2.0-2.5)
  - Malignant degeneration/progression of lower grade glioma: higher Chol/NAA ratio (>2.0-2.5)
  - Presence of lactate (1.33 ppm) in a tumor/glioma suggests necrosis and therefore higher grade.
  - Recurrent tumor (or predominantly tumor) vs radiation injury or non-neoplastic process: Cho/Cr and/or Cho/NAA ratios are higher in tumor.
- Infection:
  - Fungal infections: Trihelose peak, 3.6 to 3.8 (specific)
  - Parasitic vs pyogenic abscesses. Acetate/succinate ratio >1 in suggests pyogenic and <1 suggests parasitic.
  - Presence of glycine (3.56) peak suggests pyogenic abscess.
  - Presence of amino acids at 0.9 ppm suggests abscess/infection rather than tumor.
- Metabolic disorders:
  - Canavan disease: very high NAA, diffuse white matter signal abnormality on MRI.
  - Pelizaeus-Merzbacher disease - elevated NAA peak.
  - Salla disease - high peak at 2.03 ppm
  - Phenylketonuria - phenylalanine (7.36 ppm), can be used to follow treatment/disease progression.
  - Maple syrup urine disease - branched-chain α-keto and amino acids at 0.9 ppm
  - Mitochondrial disorders, including Leigh disease: increased lactate in brain parenchyma and possibly in ventricular CSF.
- Dementias (rarely used, unclear added value):
  - Alzheimer's disease – supported by reduced NAA/Cr ratio and elevation of Myo/Cr ratio, in paralimbic cortical regions.

  - Epilepsy:
    - Temporal lobe epilepsy - reduction in NAA concentration and NAA/(Cho + Cr) ratio correlates with side of seizure focus.

- Interpret any concurrent MRI brain in usual fashion.
  - MR spectroscopy needs to be interpreted in the context of structural MRI findings, ideally MR perfusion, and clinical context.

- Proofread your report.

References:

1. Bertholdo D, Watcharakorn A, Castillo M. Brain proton magnetic resonance spectroscopy: introduction and overview. Neuroimaging Clinics. 2013 Aug 1;23(3):359-80.
2. Sitter B, Sjøbakk TE, Larsson HB, Kvistad KA. Clinical MR spectroscopy of the brain. Tidsskrift for den Norske laegeforening: tidsskrift for praktisk medicin, ny raekke. 2019 Mar 25;139(6).
3. Öz G, Alger JR, Barker PB, Bartha R, Bizzi A, Boesch C, Bolan PJ, Brindle KM, Cudalbu C, Dinçer A, Dydak U. Clinical proton MR spectroscopy in central nervous system disorders. Radiology. 2014 Mar;270(3):658-79.
4. Gharzeddine K, Hatzoglou V, Holodny AI, Young RJ. MR perfusion and MR spectroscopy of brain neoplasms. Radiologic Clinics. 2019 Nov 1;57(6):1177-88.
5. Vachhani JA, Lee WC, Desanto JR, Tsung AJ. Magnetic resonance spectroscopy imaging characteristics of cerebral blastomycosis. Surgical neurology international. 2014;5.

MR Perfusion for Tumor

MR perfusion methods allow evaluation of cerebral blood flow, cerebral blood volume, and vascular permeability. There are several methods that can be used to measure cerebral perfusion, but most common include DSC, DCE, and ASL. In this chapter, we will discuss DSC (dynamic susceptibility perfusion imaging). These methods can differentiate high grade tumor from treatment-related changes as well as high grade glioma from metastasis and primary CNS lymphoma.

DSC perfusion imaging provides various parameters, but rCBV (corrected relative cerebral blood volume) is the most studied to assess tumors. CBF (cerebral blood flow) has similar utility in ASL (arterial spin labeled) perfusion techniques because usually lesions with increased CBV also have increased CBF.

MR perfusion is especially useful in evaluating high grade gliomas (e.g., glioblastoma) after treatment, because MR imaging can be difficult to interpret in the first 3–6 months after completion of radiation therapy and concurrent treatment with temozolomide; rCBV values can provide important information to differentiate pseudoprogression and true early progression. rCBV can also be used to differentiate true treatment response from pseudoresponse.

Calculation of rCBV is performed using manual delineation of a region of interest (ROI) on rCBV map fused with either post-gadolinium imaging sequence or FLAIR sequence. After drawing the ROI on the lesion, contralateral copy ROI can be generated to obtain normal brain rCBV values. The ratio of Tumor (T) to Normal (N), can be reported in the radiology report as T/N ratio (Figure 1). Different institutions have different cutoff values for tumor recurrence based on their individual protocols.

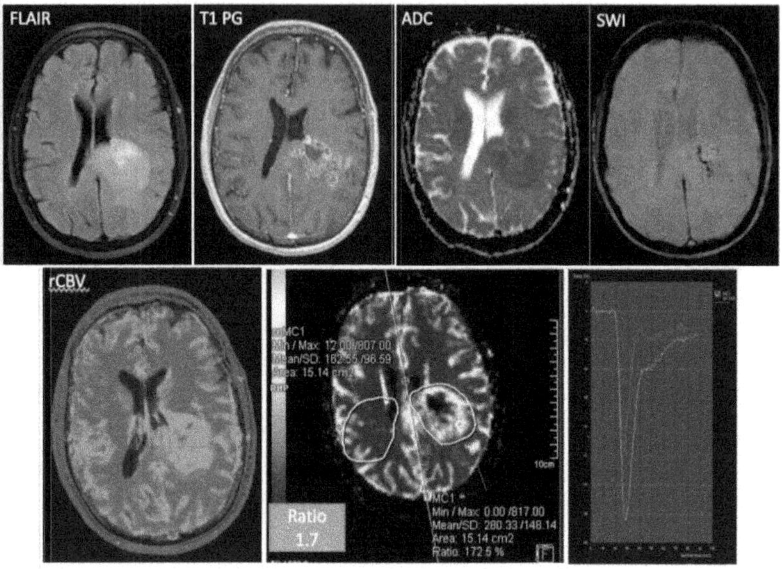

Figure 1: MRI and DSC perfusion in glioblastoma (IDH wildtype, hypermutated).

The infiltrative mass is centered within the left parietal white matter with extension into the splenium of the corpus callosum. The mass demonstrates regions of avid enhancement, necrosis, low ADC values, and minimal hemorrhage. The elevated rCBV values can be seen on rCBV map generated on either the DynaSuite software or on the SyngoVia software. The SyngoVia software was used to draw an ROI around the tumor in single plane and contralateral mirror ROI was generated. The T/N ratio was calculated to be 1.7. The signal intensity curve within the ROI was generated and area under the curve within the tumor is larger than within the normal ROI. The signal intensity curve comes close to the baseline value but does not fully reach it, which is characteristic of GBM.

Below is a "cheat sheet" for use of MR perfusion in tumor. It is not meant to be comprehensive, though represents a reasonable minimum that fellows should know before interpreting perfusion in tumor evaluation.

The broader framework for perfusion imaging of primary brain neoplasia:

- Abnormally high rCBV usually represents high grade tumor; this predicts poor outcome.
- If pursued, biopsy should be directed to high rCBV areas. It is important to describe which portion of the tumor has elevated rCBV – which portion of enhancing tumor has high rCBV and which portion of non-enhancing tumor has high rCBV.
- Low/normal rCBV usually reflects radiation necrosis/post-treatment change, or other, non-neoplastic process.
    - Compare to pre-treatment rCBV values (baseline), if lower, this favors post-treatment change.
    - Rule of thumb:
        - Low tumor blood volume (rCBV less than 1.0-1.5) indicates pseudoprogression.
        - High tumor blood volume (rCBV greater than 2.0) indicates high-grade tumor.
- rCBV values are not always low in pseudoprogression - interpret DSC perfusion in context of documented MGMT methylation status, because rCBV values in MGMT methylated tumors can have high rCBV in setting of pseudoprogression. In MGMT unmethylated glioblastomas, pseudoprogression will have low rCBV values.
- rCBV values should be reported in radiologic report and information on contralateral normal rCBV is also important. Tumor/normal ratio is a great way to report the data. rCBV values can be used for prognostication.

Most important pitfalls/exceptions to the above paradigm:

- Oligodendroglioma can have high rCBV, similar to IDH-mutant astrocytomas, even when low grade (a pitfall). Make sure you know the pathologic diagnosis of the tumor when interpreting perfusion weighted imaging in follow up cases!
- The periphery of an abscess can also have high rCBV, related to neovascularity from the immune reaction. Make sure you know the clinical setting, and correlate with conventional MRI characteristics (internal DWI signal) to assess the possibility of infection.
- Absence of abnormally high rCBV within the non-enhancing portion of the tumor does not exclude residual tumor/glioma and tumor grade affects the results. (I.e., in glioblastoma, if rCBV is low, one can say "no evidence of tumor recurrence," but in cases of low grade gliomas you cannot say that).
- Low/normal rCBV can be seen in primary CNS lymphoma (in contrast to high grade glioma).
- Interpretation of rCBV at the brain/skull base interface or near sylvian fissure can be difficult due to artifact.
- Even benign extra-axial tumors (e.g., meningiomas and schwannomas) can have higher than expected rCBV due to lack of blood brain barrier. Be sure you can localize any lesion as intra-axial or extra-axial prior to interpreting the perfusion imaging.

Differentiating high grade glioma from other entities:

- rCBV is low or normal in tumefactive demyelinating lesions.
- rCBV is frequently elevated adjacent to the tumor core of high-grade gliomas, at the surrounding T2/FLAIR abnormality (non-enhancing portion of the tumor). This is related to peritumoral infiltration with abnormal vascular supply of this nonenhancing tumor. In contrast rCBV is often *not* elevated surrounding a solitary brain metastasis, as the abnormal T2/FLAIR signal usually represents edema.
- Time-resolved perfusion imaging can also help distinguish between high grade glioma/metastasis and lymphoma, improving accuracy when combined with rCBV (Figure 2). Percentage signal recovery is critical to look at in preoperative cases, especially when trying to differentiate solitary brain metastasis from GBM.

- A perfusion signal intensity time curve will show partial return of signal to baseline in the tumor core for high grade glioma and metastasis. Partial return to baseline will also be seen in peritumor signal abnormality for high grade glioma but not metastasis.
- The signal is expected to return to and/or go above baseline for lymphoma.
- Lack of signal return to the baseline because of high vessel permeability is indicative of brain metastasis.
- This information should be correlated with other imaging characteristics.

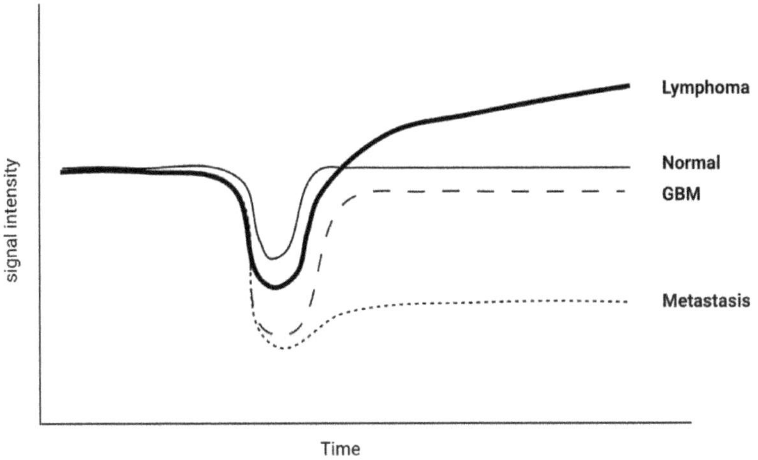

Figure 2: DSC perfusion – example of a T2* weighted signal intensity time curve for lymphoma, GBM, metastasis, and normal brain. Metastases have very strong T2* leakage effects and the signal intensity does not return to normal. GBM have mixed findings with signal between the normal and metastasis. Lymphoma has low rCBV with decreased area under the curve but the curve crosses the baseline and can keep increasing. Image created in BioRender.com.

References:

1. Jiang S, Yu H, Wang X, Lu S, Li Y, Feng L, Zhang Y, Heo HY, Lee DH, Zhou J, Wen Z. Molecular MRI differentiation between primary central nervous system lymphomas and high-grade gliomas using endogenous protein-based amide proton transfer MR imaging at 3 Tesla. European radiology. 2016 Jan;26(1):64-71.
2. Neska-Matuszewska M, Bladowska J, Sąsiadek M, Zimny A. Differentiation of glioblastoma multiforme, metastases and primary central nervous system lymphomas using multiparametric perfusion and diffusion MR imaging of a tumor core and a peritumoral zone—Searching for a practical approach. PLoS One. 2018 Jan 17;13(1):e0191341.
3. Essig M, Nguyen TB, Shiroishi MS, Saake M, Provenzale JM, Enterline DS, Anzalone N, Dörfler A, Rovira À, Wintermark M, Law M. Perfusion MRI: the five most frequently asked clinical questions. American Journal of Roentgenology. 2013 Sep;201(3):W495-510.

Checklists and Tips for Common Procedures

Long H. Tu

Sandra Abi Fadel

Michele Johnson

Introduction

The purpose of this section is to provide a thorough checklist for the most common procedures you'll encounter in diagnostic neuroradiology. These include image-guided lumbar puncture, epidural injection/blood patch, CT myelogram, and CT guided biopsy. There are many other procedures in our field, which are not described here as they are less common, and may not be applicable to the interests of most trainees. These include facet injections, vertebroplasty, angiography, and many others. For a discussion of these, I'd refer readers to any of the existing dedicated texts on interventional neuroradiology.

Fluoroscopy Guided Lumbar Puncture

Image guided lumbar puncture (LP) will be the most common procedure requested of a procedural neuroradiology service. Even though most trainees will be familiar the basic steps from intern year or exposure during residency, as a fellow, you'll likely encounter more complex and challenging cases. Below is a checklist for this common procedure. I highly recommend the article "Difficult Lumbar Puncture: Pitfalls and Tips from the Trenches" (referenced at end of section). Many steps here are drawn from this excellent review.

- Review the indication and history.
    - Make sure the study is appropriate.
        - Know if you'll need to measure opening/closing pressure.
    - Know if there are any levels of recent surgery.
    - Consider CT guidance for especially challenging anatomy.
    - Consider whether the patient will require sedation or rare cases general anesthesia.
    - Make sure all consult/pre-procedure/sedation documentation is complete. Make sure all requested lab requisition documentation is provided and appropriate.
    - Know what medications the patient is on, such as anticoagulation, or for treatment of intracranial hypertension.
    - Consider bleeding risk. At our institution we use the following thresholds for all but life-threatening cases:
        - INR <1.5.
        - PLT > 50K.
        - Hold anti-PLT and anti-coagulation medications according to SIR guidelines or institutional policy
        - PLT transfusion, FFP/Vit K can be given in emergency cases.
        - In life-threatening cases with low PLTs or coagulopathy, consider use of an introducer and thin (i.e., 25- or 27-gauge) needle.
    - As applicable: recent COVID test (72 hours).
    - Is the patient consent-able? Will they require an interpreter?
    - Is the patient NPO in case there is need for sedation?

  - If the LP is for intrathecal chemotherapy/medication, make sure the administering personnel are notified and will be present.
  - Know how much fluid you will need to remove for labs.
  - For inpatients, elderly, and others as needed, consider asking the clinical team to pre-hydrate the patient, reducing the risk of a "dry tap."

- Check prior imaging.
  - On brain imaging, make sure there's no mass, hydrocephalus, herniation, etc. that may be a contraindication.
  - On lumbar spine imaging, review and plan the access site. This can be done on CT abdomen/pelvis exams.

- Plan the approach.
  - Consider candidate levels.
    - Any bony defect/window can be used, including those produced by prior surgery (preferably remote rather than recent).
    - Avoid areas with spinal stenosis (often lower levels in adults). The most common level of degenerative change in adults is L4-L5, so it's often best to start at L2-L3 or L3-L4.
    - In children, remember the cord is lower (as low as L3), so start low, e.g., L4-L5. If you need to go higher, access the lateral third of the canal.
    - Avoid recent surgical sites, areas of active healing/granulation, and areas of possible infection.
    - Avoid post-operative collections, extensive scarring, and other subcutaneous abnormalities.
    - Avoid levels with extensive epidural fat or other pathologies which reduce the size of the CSF space in the thecal sac.
  - Measure skin to thecal sac distance. Add a few cm to get intended needle size. Note that angled approaches, mobile subcutaneous fat/tissue, and need to access a differing level if the first fails may add required length.

  - For very large/obese patients, consider an introducer (e.g., 18-gauge 1.5-inch needle). You can then use insert a smaller needle (e.g., 22 gauge) via co-axial technique. Needles are most likely to bend at the fat-muscle interface, so if you can traverse this with the introducer, you can then use the smaller needle to puncture the thecal sac.

- Pre-procedure.
  - Consent the patient.
  - Risks to communicate (uncommon/rare): bleeding, infection, nerve root injury, and post-LP headache. Advise patient to hydrate, use caffeine, rest, and contact the department (i.e., for possible blood patch) if persistent headache. Provide a contact number to the patient for issues.
  - Don't forget to ask about allergies (especially to lidocaine, or any sedation medication).
  - Make sure you have the all the appropriate LP materials opened and ready (including the correct length needle and tubing extensions for opening/closing pressure measurement).

- Position the patient on the table.
  - This procedure can be done either under conventional fluoroscopy, with a C-arm, or in an angiography room. Sterile prep may be done before or following marking of the skin puncture site.
  - Prone oblique positioning is ideal, using pillows and bent leg/arm on one side. The patient can also be placed prone/lateral decubitus, and then the C-arm rotated, as available.
  - Place a hemostat tip (or other radiopaque marker) on the patient at expected site of skin entry. Advise the patient about the imminent cold instrument touch.
  - Make sure all persons in room are leaded.

  - Check position with fluoroscopy, aiming for a "straight shot" from the skin to the thecal sac. Usually, the interlaminar space is used as a target. Reposition the marker as needed.
  - Mark the skin once satisfactory. Advise the patient that they should not move from this point forth if at all possible.
  - Don sterile gloves/gown. Prep the procedure site. Drape the patient.

- Perform a "time out."
  - Verify patient identity with two differing factors (e.g., date of birth, medical record number).
  - Verify procedure, site, and indication.
  - Note that discrepancies may be detected by any one of the care team.

- Provide local anesthesia (i.e., with 1% lidocaine without epinephrine; bicarbonate solution can be used to reduce the stinging sensation).
  - Advise the patient of impending "pinch and burning sensation."
  - Produce a wheal at the skin entry site.
  - Provide local anesthesia along intended path of needle.
  - Consider deeper anesthesia along deeper subcutaneous tissues, muscle, and periosteum. This is especially important for larger patients or for those who are at risk of moving or having greater discomfort.
  - Never use lidocaine in the LP needle!

- Insert/advance LP needle.
  - Insert as close to perfectly vertical (perpendicular to the image intensifier) as possible.
  - For larger patients, it can be useful to check the trajectory at one or two points along the length of the path to the thecal sac to make sure the needle is directed appropriately. It is much easier to correct errors in trajectory as you make the initial approach than to do so when you're already near the thecal sac.

- Bracing your hands against the patient while handling the needle can help reduce chance of inadvertent advancement if the patient moves.
- The notch at the top of the needle is same side as needle bevel; therefore, the needle will tend to move forward *away* from the notch.
- Altering the needle course can be achieved by tilting the notch/hub opposite desired tip direction. A hand at the skin surface can be a useful fulcrum.
- Another technique involves gently bending the needle at skin surface, while stabilizing the hub (a "bank shot"). This produces tip direction away for the direction of needle convexity. Be cautious of overbending when using this technique with needles less than 22-gauge.
- Advise the patient about potential for radicular pain and to speak up if this is experienced. If radicular pain is reported, stop, gently rotate your needle while checking for fluid. It may be necessary to withdraw or reposition minimally (~1mm).
- Otherwise, continue to advance until at the expected depth of the thecal sac. Advance very slowly at this depth, carefully noting any slight give/decrease in resistance. Check for fluid with each small advancement. Have a low threshold to get a lateral view.
- If you hit bone/significant resistance, withdraw minimally then check for fluid. Then check position if no fluid. If you're at the vertebral body, continue slight withdrawal and repositioning until you get CSF. If you're at a pedicle or otherwise off course, you'll have to withdraw sufficiently to be able to correct trajectory. The longer the tract and the further away from target, you more you'll have to withdraw.
- If you do not get CSF after some repositioning, a lateral view can be useful. If there is return of frank arterial/venous blood, inadvertent advancement through the disc or into the abdomen, consider terminating the procedure, and imaging for complication.
- Tilting the table, insertion and removal of the stylet, and turning the need in place can also be useful.

- If nothing gets you CSF, remember than you can:
    - Try a different lumbar level. L5-S1 is a good second choice.
    - Attempt under CT guidance, including for below.
    - Try a transforaminal approach, if other levels don't work. A full description is beyond the scope of this book, though the key point is to avoid the exiting nerve root by staying at the posterior part of the neuroforamen.
    - Try a cervical puncture as a backup (review prior images first). Again, not described fully here, but the essential detail is to stay more lateral to avoid the cord.

- Collect CSF.
    - Remember to measure opening/closing pressure if this will be required for evaluation. This should be done from the level of the heart via tube position, or via accounting for needle length. The classic measurement is done with the patient in left lateral decubitus, at the level of the left atrium.
    - Removing CSF can be a slow process. Taking too much too quickly can be associated with spinal headaches. However, if the rate of removal is painstaking, several strategies can be used to encourage flow:
        - Place the patient in reverse Trendelenburg, with a hard stop under their feet so that they do not slip/feel unstable.
        - Use longer tubing and place the end of the collection tubing below heart level.
        - Rotation of the needle (especially so that the bevel faces the head) and very slight reposition can be useful.
        - High suction using a syringe is not recommended. You can use a small (3-5cc) syringe with air gap. Provide gentle suction, including slight plunger rotation.
        - Make sure not to lose access via manipulating the spinal needle directly or via movement of the tubing.

Stabilize your needle against the patient before attaching anything to the hub.

  - Remember that depending on requested labs, cytometry, flow cytometry, differing amounts of fluid will be required.

- Post-procedure.
  - Remove the needle, bandage the patient. Have the patient remain lying down/supine for 30-60mins post-procedure.
  - Note any immediate symptoms.
  - Ensure proper label and transport of collected samples.
  - Dictate the study (and any post-procedure note).
    - Note level of access, type of needle used, and any symptoms.
    - Note fluoroscopy time, sedation dosages and duration.
    - Note amount and appearance of CSF removed.
    - Note opening CSF pressure, and position where obtained (lateral decubitus or prone).

- Proofread your dictation.

References:

1. Hudgins PA, Fountain AJ, Chapman PR, Shah LM. Difficult lumbar puncture: pitfalls and tips from the trenches. American Journal of Neuroradiology. 2017 Jul 1;38(7):1276-83.
2. Cauley KA. Fluoroscopically guided lumbar puncture. American Journal of Roentgenology. 2015 Oct;205(4):W442-50.

Lumbar Epidural Injection

This section focuses on the interlaminar approach to epidural injection. A transforaminal approach can also be used, and may be preferred for patients with unilateral symptoms or for whom an interlaminar approach is technically challenging. Caudal injection is another possibility. These procedures may be done under fluoroscopy or CT guidance.

Epidural injection is performed for patients with disc disease with or without radicular pain, spinal stenosis, axial low back pain, and recurrent symptoms after lumbar surgery. The process is very similar to the lumbar puncture, though you'll stop the needle as you enter the epidural space, rather than entering the thecal sac. A few essential notes and modifications relative to the lumbar puncture are provided below.

- Check the indication, history, and priors.
    - It is essential to know the site and type of pain. Look at prior CT/MRI studies to identify active pain generators and correlate with patient symptoms.
    - Patient interview and chart review should focus on:
        - Back versus leg/radicular predominance, dermatomal/radicular distribution.
        - Identification of any concurrent Baastrup disease, facet, or Bertolotti syndrome.
        - All imaging available in the area to evaluate accessibility.
    - Understanding whether there is correlation between symptoms and prior imaging helps you determine whether the procedure would be therapeutically successful, and/or if alternative approaches should be used.
        - Concordant symptoms, imaging findings, and accessibility should guide choice of level.
    - Note usual contraindications to spinal procedures, including coagulopathy and any contrast allergies. Consider CT guidance if the approach will be especially challenging.
        - If the patient has a contrast allergy, you can use air as contrast material under CT guidance.

- Plan the procedure, position, and prep the patient in analogous fashion as previously described for lumbar puncture (though you will target the epidural space instead).
    - A paramedian or slightly obliqued approach can be helpful to make more visible the intralaminar space.
    - Intraspinous approaches can be used in some patients.

- Remember to do a "time out."

- After local anesthesia, introduce/advance the needle until it approaches the posterior margin of the facets (estimated by length of needle and/or correlation with lateral view).

- Take the stylet out. Attach a syringe containing saline, contrast, or air.
    - Tap lightly on the plunger with one hand while advancing slowly with the other.

- Continue advancing in short increments (~1 mm) while assessing resistance to see if you've entered the posterior epidural space.
    - Lightly injecting puffs of contrast (or air) as you advance will cause the plunger to bounce back if you're outside of the epidural space. This resistance will decrease and the plunger will move forward when the needle is inside the epidural space. Be sure to advance very slowly/carefully, to avoid overshooting and entering the thecal sac.
    - If you enter the thecal sac, you must approach again from at a different location. Next level up or down is acceptable.

- Confirm location in posterior epidural space with a few cc of contrast injection. If under CT guidance, air could alternatively be used as contrast.
    - Look closely (via magnified, columnated, lateral views) for evidence of incorrect positioning. You are looking for contrast to be ill-defined and NOT outline nerve roots.
    - Intrathecal contrast injection will surround the nerve roots.
    - For patient safety, if you cannot prove that you're in epidural space, don't inject any medication.

- Inject the therapeutic mixture (preservative-free steroid, bupivacaine) into the epidural space.
    - Inject under low pressure.
    - Note any immediate symptoms.

- Recovery is similar to lumbar punctures.
    - The patient should be alerted to watch for fever, worsening focal pain, severe bruising, bleeding, or neurologic deficit.
    - Usual post procedural care: bedrest for at least 1-2 hours (optimally 24 hours post procedure) to allow for coagulation. No heavy lifting for several days. We routinely advise "nothing heavier than a gallon of milk for 5 days."

- Dictate the study (and any post-procedure note).
    - Note level of access, type of needle used, and any symptoms.
    - Note fluoroscopy time, sedation dosages and duration.

- Proofread.

References:

1. Palmer WE. Spinal injections for pain management. Radiology. 2016 Dec;281(3):669-88.
2. Shim E, Lee JW, Lee E, Ahn JM, Kang Y, Kang HS. Fluoroscopically guided epidural injections of the cervical and lumbar spine. Radiographics. 2017 Mar;37(2):537-61.
3. Roberts D, Muzio DB, et al. Lumbar interlaminar epidural injection. https://radiopaedia.org/articles/lumbar-interlaminar-epidural-injection?lang=us. Accessed 6/17/2021.

Epidural Blood Patch

Autologous epidural blood path is used to treat headaches from CSF leak, either related to dural puncture (e.g., prior LP) or spontaneous leak. The approach is nearly identical to for epidural medication injections, except that the patient's own blood is used to seal potential sites of CSF leak. Major modifications and points to keep in mind are highlighted below. For further discussion, see the provided reference which is an excellent and quick read.

- Check the indication, history, and priors.
    - Make sure the patient meets usual indications, e.g., no response to conservative treatment (rest, IV hydration, PO analgesics, IV/PO caffeine) or inability to tolerate the 7-10 days it would take for usual improvement. Make sure that there is not some other/better explanation for the patient's presentation.
    - Note that this procedure is relatively contraindicated in patients with active infection at access site, coagulopathy, allergy to utilized medications, and pregnancy. Pregnant patients could receive a non-x-ray guided blood patch.
    - Review prior imaging that might support the diagnosis, such as evidence of intracranial hypotension on MRI/CT brain, or direct evidence of leak on MR/CT myelographic studies.
    - Know what level any prior LP or other spinal procedure was done – this is where you'll target.
    - In the setting of spontaneous leak, consider obtaining imaging to look for site of leak if not previously performed.
    - Look for potential obstacles to epidural space access, specifically degenerative changes, spinal stenosis, variant anatomy, and prior surgery. Consider a CT guided approach if there is a specific site for blood patch, and access may be particularly challenging. For suspected leak that cannot be localized on imaging, you can empirically inject at L2-L3.

- Prepare the patient as usual.
    - The patient should have a peripheral IV prior to the procedure for moderate sedation. Epidural blood patch (especially with large volume injection) can be

uncomfortable, producing back pain or cramping in buttocks or thighs.
  - There should be another, sterile peripheral IV placed just before the procedure for blood draw. Confirm ability to draw blood from the IV with the patient in the position that they will be in for the blood patch.

- Plan the procedure, position, and prep the patient in analogous fashion as previously described for epidural injection and lumbar puncture.

- Remember to do a "time out."

- After local anesthesia, introduce/advance the needle until it approaches the posterior margin of the facets (estimated by length of needle and/or correlation with lateral view).

- Take the stylet out. Attach a syringe containing saline, contrast, or air.
  - Tap lightly on the plunger with one hand while advancing slowly with the other.

- Continue advancing in short increments (~1 mm) while assessing resistance to see if you've entered the posterior epidural space.
  - Lightly injecting puffs of contrast (or air) as you advance will cause the plunger to bounce back if you're outside of the epidural space. This resistance will decrease and the plunger will move forward when the needle is inside the epidural space. Be sure to advance very slowly/carefully, to avoid overshooting and entering the thecal sac.
  - If you enter the thecal sac, you must approach again from at a different location. Next level up or down is acceptable.

- Confirm location in posterior epidural space with a few cc of contrast injection. If under CT guidance, air could alternatively be used as contrast.
  - Look closely (via magnified, columnated, lateral views) for evidence of incorrect positioning. You are looking for contrast to be ill-defined and NOT outline nerve roots.

  - Intrathecal contrast injection will surround the nerve roots.
  - For patient safety, if you cannot prove that you're in epidural space, don't inject.

- Inject autologous blood, freshly drawn from the sterile IV.
  - Inject slowly to minimize patient discomfort.
  - 10-20 mL total can used for headaches after LP or similar procedures.
  - 20-50 mL total can used for spontaneous CSF leak, up to patient tolerance.
  - More than either of the above could be used in some cases.
  - A lesser amount should be used in any thoracic level injection, to avoid producing cord compression. Even 3-5 mL may be sufficient at a thoracic level if appropriately targeted.
  - The total volume injected is determined by patient comfort/tolerance. Slight Trendelenburg and slow injection can facilitate injection of greater volume.

- Recovery is similar as to for lumbar punctures.
  - The patient should be alerted to watch for fever, severe bruising, bleeding, or neurologic deficit. Advise the patient that achy back pain for several days is expected with large volume patches.
  - Usual post procedural care: bedrest for at least 1-2 hours (optimally 24 hours post procedure) to allow for coagulation. No heavy lifting for several days. We routinely advise "nothing heavier than a gallon of milk for 5 days."

- Dictate the study (and any post-procedure note).
  - Note level of access, type of needle used, and any symptoms.
  - Note fluoroscopy time, sedation dosages and duration.

- Proofread.

References:

1. White B, Lopez V, Chason D, Scott D, Stehel E, Moore W. The lumbar epidural blood patch: A Primer. Applied Radiology. 2019 Mar 1;48(2):25-30.
2. Tubben RE, Jain S, Murphy PB. Epidural blood patch. StatPearls [Internet]. 2020 Feb 10.

CT Myelogram

CT myelogram is used to evaluate intradural extramedullary lesions including cysts, webs, mass lesions, and CSF leaks; pre-myelogram LP is similar to LP for CSF collection. It's important to know if you'll want dynamic/delayed images to see communication of the thecal sac and any cystic structure or to look for subtle CSF leak or CSF-venous fistula. Note that fluoroscopic and digital images can also be helpful for diagnosis in patients with post-surgical instrumentation and patients with spondylosis and contraindication for MR imaging.

- Review the indication, history, and prior studies.
  - Make sure there is no allergy to contrast (you may need to premedicate.)
  - Consider bleeding risk. At our institution we use the following thresholds for all but life-threatening cases:
    - INR < 1.5.
    - PLT > 50K.
    - Hold anti-PLT and anti-coagulation medications according to SIR guidelines or institutional policy
    - PLT transfusion and/or FFP/Vit K can be given in emergency cases.
  - Is this study truly necessary? Can a less invasive study, such as CT, MRI or PET/CT answer the clinical question, and will any findings seen only on myelography change management?
    - Check previous imaging, as often the answer may be found on unrelated studies. Abdominopelvic imaging, may adequately demonstrate severe stenosis by disk osteophyte complex where myelography is done for spondylosis evaluation.

- Make sure you have the correct contrast for intrathecal use; concentrations differ from intravascular use.
  - E.g., Omnipaque 180, 240, and 300 may be used in adults intrathecally. Omnipaque 180 only may be used in children.
  - Do not use Omnipaque 140 or 350, which can cause seizures and other serious adverse outcomes.

- Do not forget to check the label!

- Follow the procedure for lumbar puncture as described in the prior section, up to point of the thecal sac access (CSF return).
  - Instill a small amount (1-2 mL) of contrast and confirm position by looking for flow away from needle tip (rather than pooling). Cross table lateral view can be helpful here.
  - Continue instilling contrast, looking for the expected filing defects of the cauda equina/nerve roots. Unwanted epidural injection can be identified by thin contrast circumferentially tracking into the epineural sheath.

- After instilling contrast into the thecal sac:
  - Disperse the contrast throughout the length of the thecal sac by tilting the table if needed.
  - Keep just the patient's head elevated so that contrast makes it to the cervical spine, but does not reflux into the intracranial compartment (unless looking for skull base pathology).
  - To get contrast to flow superiorly, turn the patient lateral oblique. Contrast can flow up the thoracic kyphosis more easily via the lateral gutter of the thecal sac, and with a lesser curvature in the direction of gravity. You'll likely still need to tilt the table in a craniocaudal direction, but you might then require less angulation.
  - If there is a level of severe spinal canal stenosis, consider flexion or extension in whichever direction straightens out/improves patency of the spinal canal at that level.

- CT image acquisition:
  - The patient should be immediately transported to the CT scanner.
  - Have the patient turn over several (e.g., three) times just prior to performing the CT study to avoid contrast layering.
  - Consider dual energy CT and metallic hardware artifact reduction as needed to visualize the thecal sac.

    - Scan at a delayed time point when there is concern for CSF leak or to characterize connection of any cyst with the thecal sac.

- Recovery is similar as to for LPs.

- Interpret the study in similar fashion as usual CT/MRI studies.
    - Note level of access, type of needle used, and any symptoms with thecal sac access.
    - Note fluoroscopy time, sedation dosages and duration.

- Proofread.

References:

1. Patel DM, Weinberg BD, Hoch MJ. CT myelography: clinical indications and imaging findings. Radiographics. 2020 Mar;40(2):470-84.
2. Pomerantz SR. Myelography: modern technique and indications. Handbook of clinical neurology. 2016 Jan 1;135:193-208.
3. OMNIPAQUE™ (iohexol) Injection. https://www.accessdata.fda.gov/drugsatfda_docs/label/2017/018956s099lbl.pdf. Accessed 9/19/2021.

CT Guided Spine/Soft Tissue Biopsy

After image guided lumbar-puncture, the most commonly requested procedure we do is CT guided biopsy of spinal and paraspinal lesions. Depending on the institution, you may also sample sacral, facial, and other head and neck lesions. Many of the concepts covered here apply to CT guided biopsy in general, and form a basis for these other sites.

Here, we discuss sampling in the thoracic and lumbar spine. We use a trans-pedicular approach whenever possible. Extra-pedicular/posterolateral and trans-costovertebral are other options, and may be useful for predominately paraspinal abnormalities. A complete discussion of these techniques is beyond the scope of this book; however, they are discussed more fully in the provided references.

Below is an outline our process for CT guided biopsy of (thoracolumbar) spinal lesions.

- Check the indication, history, and any prior studies.
    - Is the biopsy necessary? Is there a better/safer/less invasive target than what was requested? Will this change management?
    - Know what the clinical suspicion for underlying pathology is, including whether it includes infection, lymphoma, other metastatic/neoplastic etiologies. Be sure not to biopsy vascular lesions/malformations by accident.
        - In setting of infection, consider if currently drawn blood cultures could yield a diagnosis without need for invasive procedure.
    - Is the patient consent-able? Will they require an interpreter?
    - Is the patient NPO if there is need for sedation?
    - Is there any reason this patient might need general anesthesia rather than just moderate sedation and local anesthesia (e.g., not able to cooperate or tolerate procedure otherwise?)
    - Make sure to check prior imaging to make sure you know what you're going after and that it is feasible. Sometimes a review of the history/imaging can make it clear the biopsy should not be performed.
        - Consider reviewing key prior studies as seriously as if you were reporting the study yourself. Reach out

to the clinical team if you have an opinion differing from to the official report.

- Plan your approach:
  - In the lumbar spine, avoid a path that is in line with the aorta, IVC, and iliac vessels. For paraspinal masses, avoid a path that includes the renal vessels or kidneys.
  - In the thoracic spine, if using a superior or inferior costovertebral approach, angle anteromedially to avoid the pleura, and stay just above the rib to avoid the intercostal nerve and vessels.
  - Decide how you'll position the patient: prone, oblique, or lateral decubitus and feet or head first. Very obese patients may have difficulty breathing while prone, so consider lateral decubitus. Positioning can aid in ease of access to the lesion otherwise.
  - Chose a path that would allow sampling of both osseous and soft tissue components if both are present in an abnormality.
  - Measure the length of the expected path to the lesion.
  - Measure the distance between the skin and any bony cortex you'll traverse, as well as between the skin and the lesion. Also measure from the skin to any vital structures on the other side of planned approach. Pick a needle length that would make it difficult/impossible to go too deep and injure major structures on the other side.
  - If you'll traverse a pedicle, make sure it is sufficiently wide/positioned to accommodate the path of your needle without fracture of the medial or lateral cortices.
- Consider bleeding risk. At our institution we use the following thresholds for all but life-threatening cases:
  - INR < 1.5.
  - PLT > 50.
  - Hold anti-PLT and anti-coagulation medications according to SIR guidelines or institutional policy.

        - Consider systemic coagulopathies (DIC, von Willibrands disease, hemophilias, etc).
        - Check renal function if the lesion needs to be scanned with contrast.
    - Make sure any pre-procedure charting/notes are done.
        - Pre-procedure/consult note.
        - Moderate sedation.
        - Consent.
        - As applicable: recent COVID test (72 hours).
    - Make sure you have the correct solutions for the type of biopsy.
        - Formalin is used for most things.
        - Saline is required if the pathologists will do frozen sections for a preliminary read.
        - You'll need a special solution if there is any concern or lymphoma (e.g., RPMI).

- Time out and grid placement.
    - Make sure you have a mask, cap, and gown as needed.
    - Do a time out.
    - Get localizer images.
    - Pick a potential window/table position around the expected site of the lesion. Position patient at the chosen table position.
    - Double check the representation of the patient on the scanning computer. Clarify to yourself which side of the table/patient is which side of the image. The orientation changes based on which way the patient is facing and if they are feet or head first into the scanner.
    - For lesions which might move with respirations, the patient should be asked to breath-hold during planning scans and biopsy, to reproduce as close the same positioning as possible.
    - Attach the grid to patient at the skin position of expected entry to the lesion.
    - Scan the patient. Adjust the table position as needed. Angling the table is an option on some scanners.

- Prep and provide local anesthesia.
    - Choose your approach and mark the patient's skin at the grid position where you'll enter. It's best to mark with an "X" (i.e., two intersecting lines) rather than a single line or dot, which can be easily smudged, confusing the skin target.
    - Remove the grid.
    - Don sterile gloves (with or without gown depending on infection risk).
    - Prep and drape the patient.
    - Administer local anesthetic, using the anesthetic needle to plan the angle of approach. It can be useful to anesthetize deeply, along the expected course of the needle. Aspirate before injection to make sure you're not injecting intravascularly.
    - Scan the patient around the entry site.

- Approach the lesion with a guide needle.
    - Perform a small skin incision for the needle.
    - Insert the guide needle at the position/angle to approach the lesion. Depending on the thickness of the subcutaneous tissues, it can be useful go a third to a half the distance to the lesion (or overlying cortex, if a bone lesion) on the first pass. Subcutaneous fat is more mobile (and less vascular) than muscle, so if there is significant thickness to traverse, consider a pause/check prior to entering muscle.
    - The deeper you are, the harder it as to change trajectory.
    - Rescan around the needle to check position. Correct angle and/or translate the needle in space as needed.
    - Repeat continual adjustment and advancement until you're at bone on a trajectory that is headed to the preferred region of the target lesion.
    - Infiltrating the paraspinal muscles and spinal periosteum with local anesthetic can reduce patient discomfort and make the procedure go more smoothly.

- Drill through bone (for osseous lesions).
    - This can be done with a manual or electric drill depending on your biopsy kit.
    - Place the drill bit through the guide needle and continue advancing the drill and then the guide needle behind it as you approach the lesion. Be careful of osteoporotic or otherwise

abnormal bone. Unexpected drops in resistance can make you advance further than you intend.
  - Check the scans intermittently so that you know when you are at the edge of the lesion. It can be useful to stop just before you traverse the last of normal bone. Having normal bone on the edge of the sample allows the pathologist to assess the margin of the sample with normal tissue.
  - Scan one last time prior to performing the biopsy, with the guide needle positioned just before the site where you want to sample. On the workstation images, measure to ensure that the additional length of biopsy would not pass into another structure. The additional length beyond the guide needle can be adjusted with some kits.

- Sample the lesion.
  - Insert the biopsy needle. You may have to push/turn the needle through resistance if the lesion retains some bony structure.
  - Scan/obtain images to document position of needle in the lesion.
  - If possible, sample the periphery of the lesion at the transition from normal bone. Avoid central necrotic or cystic areas.
  - Remove the biopsy needle and split the sample as needed for differing tests.
  - We usually do 2-3 core biopsies for osseous lesions. Soft tissue components are sampled simultaneously. You can biopsy the soft tissue component of a lesion that has complete replaced bone with a dedicated kit.
  - An aspirate is obtained after cores, if possible.

- Post-procedure.
  - If you suspect the lesion to be hypervascular, consider a scan of the patient prior to removing the needle. Excessive local bleeding can be controlled by gelfoam along the needle tract.
  - Remove the needles. Clean and bandage the patient.
  - Obtain post-biopsy images to look for hematoma or other complication (if not already obtained).
  - Start discharge/transfer, pathology, and relevant nursing orders.

  - Observation time after procedure depends on how much sedation was given. Warn the patient to watch for fever, severe bruising, bleeding, or neurologic deficit. Provide pain control/prescription as needed.
  - Print any requisition forms you'll need to send with the sample.
  - Write any required brief procedure note and dictate the study.
  - Note radiation dose as well as dosages of moderate sedation provided.

- Proofread your dictation.

References:

1. Saifuddin A, Palloni V, du Preez H, Junaid SE. the current status of CT-guided needle biopsy of the spine. Skeletal Radiology. 2020 Aug 19:1-9.
2. Peh WC. CT-guided percutaneous biopsy of spinal lesions. Biomedical imaging and intervention journal. 2006 Jul;2(3).

Workflow and Team Efficiency Tips

Long H. Tu

Kimberly Seifert

Anthony Abou Karam

Introduction

Individual efficiency is just one part of the picture in having a successful fellowship experience. If you are working as part of a team with both residents and fellows, there are numerous ways to optimize the workflow. This presumes you/your program leadership have some control over the work organization.

Most of what is discussed here has been implemented at the authors' programs. The motivation in recounting these efforts is to share insights which may similarly improve work experience elsewhere. I have to reiterate that while multiple people contributed thoughts to this writing, I (L.T.) am ultimately responsible for opinions expressed here.

Communication Triage and Automation

Phone Trees and Radiology Assistants

For a busy neuroradiology services, the number of phone calls, consults, protocol requests and other interruptions to the interpretive workflow can be overwhelming. At the beginning of my fellowship year, approximately 50% of the phone calls to the main reading room were ultimately redirected to a differing part of the neuroradiology "team" – whether the procedure service, technologists, schedulers, or CT/other reading rooms, etc. The implementation of a phone tree (in collaboration with hospital telecom) was able to almost completely eliminate unnecessary calls, and cut total call volume by ~50%.

In some departments, the hiring of a "radiology assistant" or "phone triage" staff to help manage calls is another incredibly effective means of minimizing interruptive non-interpretive work. For off hours, some of these responsibilities can be turned into resident moonlighting opportunities. Staff filling this role help contact clinical staff with critical results and coordinates incoming calls to the appropriate radiology personnel. This sort of aid does not just make communication more efficient. It profoundly improves the quality of work life and can ameliorate some of the worst contributors to burnout. Reducing interruptions can also improve patient care by protecting against diagnostic error that arises from disrupted interpretive work.

Digital Communication

The most common non-emergent communications we had in our fellowship were requests for protocols, to QA studies, and to approve requests for urgent outpatient imaging. The advent of a text "communicator" as part of the PACS allowed technologists to contact the designated radiologist (consult fellow) unobtrusively rather than calling the room. This dramatically reduced phone call interruptions. The use of a designed (HIPAA compliant) smart phone or another message application can also be useful. Use of automated/back-end systems (e.g., Veriphy) to contact clinical staff with critical or unexpected results also profoundly improves the efficiency of care.

Maximizing Preliminary Report Use

For all emergency, inpatient, and urgent outpatient imaging, releasing preliminary reports as soon as possible, and for as any cases as feasible can improve the efficiency of clinical care. Optimizing use of preliminary reporting can also reduce the number of phone calls to the reading room looking for a "wet read" or an "ETA" on studies without a final interpretation. A similar efficiency gain can be found even in pre-empting phone calls even "routine" outpatient studies, when there is an office visit where care decisions depend on the imaging results. Our PACS/workflow manager allows flagging of "appointment dependent" as a priority designation similar to "STAT" or "Urgent." Providing preliminary reports on these studies can similarly produce efficiency gains.

Preliminary report use requires a few caveats, with feasibility depending on institution and setting. While it allows a certain degree of resident/fellow autonomy, preliminary reports should only be done when a trainee is confident in their interpretation. There should be institutional buy-in and understanding that only final reports should be used for *irreversible* management decisions. Preliminary reports should contain a clear disclaimer marking them as "in progress" and stating that final report may differ significantly.

Discrepancies with the final report should be communicated by phone or automated system. With proper safety mechanisms, the use of this sort of communication can significantly improve not just patient care, but the satisfaction of referring clinicians and patients for prompt triage and report categorization, (i.e., likely normal, abnormal, or emergent.)

Protocoling Automation and Efficiency

Our institution has been able to create mechanisms where certain studies are automatically protocolled, without need for physician input. We created specific orders for referring clinical services with one-to-one correspondence to a protocol for the most common types of exams, e.g., non-contrast CT heads, "MR Brain MS" for multiple sclerosis patients, and non-contrast MRI for cord compression. This allows automation of protocol choice for instances where review by a radiologist rarely adds value and may in some cases delay care. Ability to produce such efficiencies depends on department/institutional buy-in, but can be incredibly time and effort saving where possible.

Training of radiologist assistants to do basic protocolling has helped improve efficiency in some settings. Batching of protocol responsibilities into moonlighting work (e.g., for residents), remote shifts, and during downtime in advanced MRI processing/monitoring and other rotation are other avenues that have proved fruitful.

Differentiation of Clinical Roles

Consult and Volume Roles

We have experimented with many ways to organize the fellow workflow and have found the below useful. Please note that such organization may not work for all practice settings or programs.

If you're working on a team of two or more fellows it may be more efficient to differentiate into specific tasks. Designation of one "consult" fellow to be responsible for phone calls, consults, and other small tasks helps shield other team members from interruptions. This person would not primarily be responsible for cleaning the list. The other "volume" fellow(s) could read studies uninterrupted, and carry the responsibility of managing the list. The volume fellow would only speak to clinical staff when there are questions about a case this fellow has read. Otherwise, this person never picks up the phone. Such a team may swap roles in the middle of any shift to keep things even between "consult" and "volume" roles (or scheduling can keep this fair on a larger scale).

Contrast the efficiency of differentiated roles to the less organized approach found in many reading rooms. Without clear roles, it's unclear who should pick up the phone or consult with clinicians. Calls are passed around until they get to the right person (instead of being consolidated into one person). Multiple people may try to respond to a consult or phone call at once. In some cases, no one may be available for urgent consult, if all already involved in longer cases. Many of these efficiencies can be removed via a simple differentiation of responsibilities.

Dynamic Staffing to Volume Needs

This book was written during a fellowship year that occurred wholly during a global pandemic. Our program had also acquired new imaging volume related to hospital expansion and acquisitions. Attending level staffing had undergone some unexpected changes in part related to the pandemic.

We found that the existing fellow staffing paradigm could no longer safely cover the volume required during evening/late hours and weekends, even though there was robust even extra coverage for regular hours. Few people want to work the off hours, so we attached extra time off ("post-call" or "compensation" days) for doing odd shifts. We used a similar paradigm for the weekends. This ended up smoothing out coverage gaps nicely, and made off-hour shifts more popular than even the regular ones.

Until this change, some shifts were too "easy" and others were so "hard" as to be unsafe. If you have any control or say in how staffing is done, consider relatively rapid response to changes in volume around the clock, with sufficient incentive that these changes are welcomed by all involved. Often times, it is the people doing the actual work (fellows!) who will be most affected or most in tune with shifting needs in staffing. Do not hesitate to do what is needed to improve your own experience and the safety/efficiency of the care you provide.

Differentiation of Administrative Roles

Chief Fellows and Second Year Fellows

Depending on the size of the program, it can be useful to designate specific administrative roles, to share the responsibility. For programs with 2-year fellows, those in the second year can be differentiated into roles for scheduling, coordinating lectures/didactic, and other administrative duties. Implement one or more "chief fellow" positions is one way to consolidate these roles for larger one-year fellowships. Bundling administrative work for those who have the motivation and organizational skills to manage it (and then giving them some time to fulfill those responsibilities) can help make sure that a program continues to run smoothly. This can work better than dispersing responsibilities to those without inherent interest.

Off Cycle Fellows

Off cycle fellows are those that start at a slight delay compared to the usual July 1st beginning of the hospital year. The stagger in start time may be a month or more. At our program we have at least two off cycle fellows in a group of 12. Each year, 2-3 fellows start late and end late, overlapping with the next class. The off-cycle fellows assume administrative duties (as off-cycle chief) at the beginning of the new year, passing on training and wisdom to the rising chiefs and other fellows.

The overlap is an incredible mechanism to ensure that new fellows have help onboarding and learning the ropes from trainees who are experienced. This may occur more naturally in two-year fellowships, but for 1-year only fellowships, the staggering of start times ensures a smoother transition, and a more robust retainment of program-specific knowledge about how to optimize the workflow. Even though the implementation of such a system would not immediately benefit a fellowship group the first year it is employed, the initiative to create such a system pays recurring large dividends.

Teaching and Academics

Academic Time

Fellowship classes are generally large enough to accommodate vacation, sick/personal time, and other time away. In the same way, there are potential efficiency and long-term gains to be made by scheduling "academic" time for either interested fellows, or even better, *all* fellows. Such an initiative, especially if the degree of allowance is dependent on productivity, is a means of improving academic output at a program. Especially during periods where a fellowship might be robustly or even over-staffed, providing a freedom to work on non-clinical projects allows the same amount of clinical work to be done (just bundled more efficiently) while producing meaningful contributions of a different kind.

Academic time can used to support research ventures, and launch investigations that are carried into later attending positions. Academic time could also be used to attended national conferences, participate in more than usual tumor boards/interdisciplinary conferences, or engage in quality improvement initiatives that make an enduring contribution to the program.

Efficiency Gains from Teaching

One of the most powerful, yet underutilized means of helping get the work done is to engage in teaching. If the workload is shared among residents and fellows, note that rapidly getting new residents on service up to speed with basics can pay large dividends in their work output over the course of a rotation, and ultimately over the whole year. In any case, as a fellow, you benefit from the teaching efforts of prior years' fellows (as well as residents and faculty) who have previously invested in teaching efforts for trainees who return much better situated. Consider engaging in the following highest-impact teaching and orientation activities, whether in a structured/recurring way, or opportunities arise.

Teach a crop of residents new to the service a basic approach/search pattern any of the most common exams:

- CT head
- CT cervical/thoracic/lumbar spine
- CTA head and neck
- MRI brain
- MRI cervical/thoracic/lumbar spine

CT head and MRI brain especially make up a large proportion of studies on service. Teaching any of the above may take 15-30 minutes at most, but if they make any resident even 10-20% faster for their time on service, this amounts to hours of improved study throughput over the course of a rotation. Junior residents may reasonably begin with more basic studies and pathology, meaning that as a higher-level trainee, you can focus more on complex studies and exam types.

Other high yield activities in this vein include making sure all rotating residents have efficiency-oriented macros/templates and know the best resources to learn neuroradiology. Residents should be reminded that they are responsible to share phone calls/consultation, as well as study volume. The inclusion of rotating trainees, even other fellows on elective, into the workflow increases the chances that the shared work is reasonably divided, and that everyone has a good experience.

While I've mostly commented here on the teaching of more junior trainees, it can also be incredibly helpful to engage in fellow-to-fellow or shared teaching. The sharing of workflow tips, the best way to hang/approach complex studies, hotkeys and special functionality specific to the dictation software, PACS, or institution can pay huge dividends especially at the beginning of the year. The faster and better your group of fellows is, the faster you'll progress in your education, and the faster you'll move through each day's work. In the best of circumstances, this can free up additional attending time/effort to address questions, teach, or for the best of team players – even help primarily "clean the list." Sharing of interesting cases through a case conference, a case file, or other means enhances everyone's education for less overall investment than routine practice.

Group-cohesion, educational reinforcement for the teacher, and other benefits aside, the enormous productivity return of investment on teaching means that it is a crucial activity for group efficiency. At the very least, consider engaging the highest-yield teaching activities described in this section.

Consider Leaving a Legacy

Many of the efforts that keep our program running were produced by past fellows. These include focused manuals for post-processing software, guides to the electronic medical record/PACS, and other institution-specific tips. There are also innumerable workflow optimizations, specialized macros, and teaching case collections. We would not be functional as a clinical service without these resources. Enduring contributions can be even more efficient than-on the fly, in-person teaching. Filling practical needs early in the fellowship is not just a way to "pay it forward"; it can be a way to optimize the experience during your own time. Consider leaving a legacy early on.

Conclusion

Last Comments & Contact

This book has been somewhat of memoir of my time as a fellow – the pitfalls, unwritten rules, and hard-won wisdom collected along the way. Thank you for reading this far. I hope that my co-authors and I have been able to distill the best and the most universal guidance into a form that you've found useful.

Because of its somewhat informal nature, I must again apologize for any imperfections or omissions made in the text. While the writing has been reviewed by multiple contributors and checked against the literature, I know that subtle error can be difficult to stamp out entirely. For feedback and suggestions for future editions, please consider emailing me at long.tu@yale.edu. It would be great to hear from you!

Lastly, I have to give credit to the many true experts and pioneers in our field whose original work I have referenced here. Our practice of neuroradiology would not be possible without their efforts. This guide is written out of a similar impulse to make things better. I hope in a small way, it can inspire you to also continue this tradition.

Long H. Tu

www.ingramcontent.com/pod-product-compliance
Ingram Content Group UK Ltd.
Pitfield, Milton Keynes, MK11 3LW, UK
UKHW021251190125
4172UKWH00026B/319

9 798524 122469